INTERMITTENT FASTING 16/8

The Ultimate Guide To Cleanse Your Body The Easy Way. A Simple, Safe and Sustainable Way to Lose Weight, Enhance Longevity and Improve Your Health with Minimal Effort

GEENA MOORE

DISCLAIMER

This book is meant for educational and information purposes only. It is not meant to give any medical advice, diagnose, or treat any medical conditions. No medical claims are made in this book. The nutritional advice given in this book will not treat or cure medical conditions, metabolic disorders, or other illnesses. The nutritional advice is meant for healthy individuals who want to improve their appearance for cosmetic reasons and not to treat illnesses of any kind.

You should always consult your physician or other healthcare provider should you have any questions regarding a medical condition or treatment plan.

The author is not a MD or RD and cannot be held liable or responsible to any person or entity with respect to any information contained in this book. The reader/ user assumes all risks for any injury, loss or damage caused or alleged to be caused directly or indirectly by using the information contained in this book.

Table of Contents

Introduction

Intermittent fasting is for one and all. Anyone willing to lose weight and live a healthy life is right for intermittent fasting. It is well suited for women who want to shed those extra pounds and reach fitness goals because a woman's health and body go through hills and valleys as they age. Right from the time a girl reaches maturity, marriage, pregnancy, childbirth, breastfeeding, and weaning, her body undergoes a myriad of changes. And a woman with multiple children has experienced this change and shift many times, requiring specific work to see any improvement. It is a huge testament to the wonder of nature, witnessing what a woman's body and mind can do.

In all this, if a lady wishes to lose weight, get her body back in shape, and generally remain in good health, then there can be no better way to succeed than by following an intermittent fasting pattern, especially on the 16/8 schedule. The flexibility alone makes it a perfect fit by easily accommodating the challenges of a woman's rigorous home and work life.

For someone who has never fasted before, the prospect of going without food for sixteen straight hours can seem daunting and impossible to accomplish. Many enthusiastic intermittent fasters begin their fasting journey with a bang and will fizzle out of both enthusiasm, energy and just can't seem to do it. The reason is their rush to start fasting and seeing results over a few days. Intermittent fasting is indeed fruitful, and it will bring you solid results within a short period. But the key lies in how you ease into the fasting schedule. One might assume that going without food or drinks is easy. They'll jump right into a fasting method and even find the first two days a breeze to accomplish. But on the third day is when reality kicks in and they find themselves wishing to go back to normal eating patterns and leaning toward breaking their fasts midway. What they do not realize, is what sustained them the first two days was simply adrenaline rush and excited enthusiasm. Once that drains off, they are bereft of anything driving their fasts.

Intermittent fasting is not that difficult and need not be that intimidating. What is essential is to gradually ease yourself into the fasting schedules and let your body get used to fasting periods slowly. We will now look at the different steps you can take to start your intermittent fasting journey smoothly and carry on without a hitch.

Begin with the right mindset.When you decide to try the 16/8 fasting schedule or any intermittent fasting technique for that matter, prepare yourself mentally first. Be clear about your goals and talk to yourself about what you wish to achieve through this fasting experience. Many times, weight loss simply cannot be achieved by just diet control or exercise. Combining it with the right mindset and intention is the way to begin and finish strong. Diet and exercise will only take you so far. Even if you see results, these will only be temporary as you are not touching on the root cause for weight gain in the first place.

Fat buildup can happen for many different reasons. Fat stores energy for dire need situations. Beyond this, fats perform other functions too, like offering protection and insulation from the outside world. To understand the reason for this, you might have to look deeper into your mind and look for feelings and thoughts that indicate you are anxious, scared, or in fear of something specific. We all have fears and feel threatened from time to time for different reasons we can't always explain. Our body works for us, not against us, and tries to offer some protection with layers of fat because that is its purpose.

Once you have readied yourself mentally, then the next step is to slowly transition yourself from your previous lifestyle and eating habits to newer healthier ones. Begin by making note of an average eating day for you. It is a great idea to start a food journal to record your experiences and other occurrences that stand out on your journey with intermittent fasting.

Start by recording your regular eating schedules with your mealtimes.Include any specific snack times you regularly have, any regular drinking like coffee, tea, soda, or juice. Also, include any supplements you take on a regular basis. Through all this data you will be able to chart out your plan and schedule your fasting hours to best accommodate your regular needs.

Intermittent fasting will naturally bring a huge change in your eating patterns. But, in the beginning, it is best to keep these changes to a minimum so your transition into fasting is not sudden or abrupt making it easier to handle, both mentally and physically.

This slow buildup to the sixteen-hour fast will allow your body to adjust to the rigorous schedule gradually. You will need this adjustment window to let yourself feel at ease with the demands of fasting both physically and emotionally. Continue to journal your experiences as you fast each day. Write down what you feel as your fasting hours go by. Are you excited, hungry, bored, lazy or energetic?Or see no change; keep a record of it all. This will help you look back and see what worked and what didn't. Such as which food supported your fasts and which made you hungry sooner; what activities were doable and what seemed stressful? Keeping a record of these little things will strengthen your groundwork as you move along your fasting journey. Also, journaling gives you an outlet for your emotions and will motivate yourself to continue when you feel down physically or in spirit. Personally, my journal was a huge support system on its own for me during my journey of intermittent fasting.

Intermittent fasting doesn't really dictate what you eat, it simply tells you when to eat. This, of course, does not mean you eat whatever you like and feel no consequences of your choices. Instead, you need to find the right balance between what is healthy and what is an indulgence. You don't have to give up the comfort food you love, let your favorites be 20 percent of your whole meal plan while eighty percent of caloric intake consists of healthy food. Work out how you would like this to play out. Would you prefer a serving of your favorite every three days or save it for the weekend? The bottom line is do not let intermittent fasting stop you from eating what you enjoy. Eat whatever you want, but always in moderation. Remember, the point here is to navigate the health world with positivity and happiness, and denying yourself what you love will not result in contentment. In my opinion, the 16/8 fasting schedule is the best intermittent fasting choice you can make. By simply approaching it with the right attitude and working around your own emotions and preferences can go a long way in determining how successful your fasting experience can be.

The 16/8 method is a very convenient, sustainable, and easy way in which you can easily lose weight, improve your health, and also burn fat. Also, this is often regarded as the most common style of fasting today. While all other forms of diet involve very strict rules along with regulations regarding what you can eat and what you cannot, the 16/8 method is much easier to follow. This is mainly because of its less restrictive nature, along with more flexibility when compared with other nature of diet plans. The 16/8 intermittent fasting can provide you with the best results and that too, with the minimum efforts.

While following this method, you need to complete having all your meals within a particular time period of 8 hours every day and then fast for the rest of the 16 hours each day. It depends on you how frequently you would like to repeat the cycle of fasting and eating in a week. Relying on your own choice, you can either opt for it for one time or two times a week or you can also carry on with it every day. This method will not only help you to lose weight, but it also comes with the added benefit of improving the levels of blood sugar, enhances your longevity, and also boosts up the functioning of the brain.

For starting with this method, you will first need to select a window of eight hours and then restrict all the food consumption for that period of time. For finding the best window, you can experiment with different time frames and then select the one that matches perfectly with your routine or schedule. Regardless of the food type that you have every day, it is always better for you if you have several small-sized meals along with snacks evenly distributed throughout the course of the day. This will help you a lot in controlling the hunger along with the stabilization of the level of blood sugar. For maximizing the benefits of this plan, it is very important to consume only nutritious forms of whole food along with beverages during the window of eating. When you consume foods rich in nutrients, you will be able to round up your entire diet and reap all the prizes that this diet regimen has to offer you.

You can balance your meal by having various types of whole foods. You can try various types of foods, like:

1. Proteins: Fish, meat, eggs, poultry, seeds, legumes, nuts, etc.

2. Whole grains: Quinoa, barley, rice, oats, buckwheat, etc.

3. Healthy fats: Olive oil, avocado, coconut oil, etc.

4. Vegetables: Broccoli, tomatoes, cauliflower, cucumber, green leafy vegetables, etc.

5. Fruits: Oranges, bananas, apples, peaches, berries, pears, etc.

Chapter 1 –Basic Mechanisms and Advantages of 16/8

Intermittent fasting techniques, including the 16/8 method, are most commonly used to assist in weight loss by the general population. The method has been tried by thousands of people and also scientifically proven to be a helpful resource in reducing body fat and improving body composition. Weight loss is often considered the number one reason why people opt for a diet and a program that utilizes the intermittent fasting.

While a reduction in body fat is definitely one of the best advantages to be mentioned in terms of intermittent fasting, there are more advantages that people gain—especially if they are truly commited to it and can implement self-control that ensures they do not give in to cravings.

Intermittent fasting is known to assist in improving your body composition as well, as I mentioned earlier. Body composition refers to a series of features—this includes your body fat percentage and lean muscle mass primarily. A program that utilizes intermittent fasting, along with an appropriate diet plan, will bring down your body fat percentage, and push up your lean muscle mass at the same time.

It is also important to note the benefits associated with weight loss for people with an excessive amount of fat distributed throughout their bodies. Since overweight and obesity are linked to so many chronic conditions that can truly make your life dreadful, losing even small amounts of weight can drastically reduce your risk of these diseases. Additionally, if you already have a diagnosis of a condition associated with obesity, reduced body weight may improve the symptoms you are experiencing and help you get the disease under control.

In turn, these things all have factors that link them to insulin resistance. When insulin resistance develops, it can continue to progress into type 2 diabetes if the affected person does not implement appropriate preventive measures.

When you develop type 2 diabetes, you become predisposed to many additional risks and complications. In fact, type 2 diabetes can cause severe complications that may not only lead to disability but also become life-threatening. This disease can also affect all of the body's most important organs, including the heart, and can damage various tissues, such as nerves, throughout the body.

In addition to assisting in reducing body weight and bringing down the risks associated with obesity, intermittent fasting has many other benefits that are also worth mentioning.

Through intermittent fasting, cellular changes may occur in the body. This can lead to levels of human growth hormones rising by as much as 500%. This leads to a faster rate of fat burning while also producing an increase in muscle mass.

It has also been found that intermittent fasting can help to remove waste that has built up in cells within the human body and can also assist in the repair process of cells that have been damaged. This means cells in the body become more efficient in performing their specialized functions.

One study also explains how recent findings from scientists suggest that intermittent fasting helps to improve brain health and may play a crucial role in assisting medical experts in understanding better how diseases like Parkinson's disease and Alzheimer's disease can be prevented in the future.

Furthermore, following an intermittent fasting plan can also help to reduce levels of inflammation within the human body, as well as help to fight against oxidative stress. Both of these factors are known to contribute to numerous chronic diseases significantly and can cause certain molecules to become damaged, which can inhibit their functionality within the body.

In one study, scientists tested how intermittent fasting would work on brain health and cardiovascular health among a group of laboratory rats. They found significant improvements in various tests used to determine the well-being of these two crucial hormones of the body. The scientists also associated these improvements among the tested laboratory rats with a reduction in oxidative stress that was observed.

Additionally, the scientists also found an increase in the cellular stress resistance ratings in these rats. What this means is that an intermittent fasting diet can help to reduce the effect stress has on the body, and help to fight against the existing oxidative damage, often also referred to as free radical damage that has already occurred.

Intermittent Fasting Different Models and 16/8:

With the core concept out of the way, the next thing that I believe you should know about is the different types of intermittent fasting protocols that are available to you.

Yes, you heard that right!

There's much more to intermittent fasting than just stopping to eat and eating again when the right time comes.

Due to the demands and physiological conditions of different human beings, scientists and nutritionists have crafted out a number of different types of intermittent fasting protocols.

Each of these different types of protocols is designed to cater to a specific type of audience.

While there are lots of different programs, below are some of the core ones that you should know about.

Spontaneous Meal Skip:

This protocol does not come packed with a specific fasting period and rather works on giving you the freedom to choose your very own time frame.

This means if one fine morning you don't feel hungry, you can simply skip breakfast on that morning and fast till dinner and have a healthy meal to top it off. Alternatively, you may also skip lunch and dinner and have breakfast!

The whole point of the protocol is to give you the freedom to make your fasting routine.

Alternatively, you may also opt to skip lunch and dinner and breakfast altogether. The whole point of this plan is to allow you to make the most perfect and beneficial plan for you.

The Warrior Diet:

This particular program was created by one expert known as Ori Hofmekler and according to him, the best way of fasting is to expose yourself to as many vegetables and fruits as possible.

Keeping that in mind, Ori moved forward with his particular plan that further inspired people to eat very little portions of vegetables and fruits throughout the whole day and making sure to end the day with a nice and hearty meal.

After dinner, you are required to completely fast for 4 hours at least and continue the cycle once again.

Alternate Day Method:

This particular method will require you to simply fast for any particular day and then choose to skip fasting the next day. To make things clearer, if you fast the whole day today, you are allowed to skip fasting for the next day.

The thing about this that you should know is that there are actually a number of different variations of this particular protocol. So, make sure to do your research and choose the one that suits you. Regardless, the main aim of all the protocols is to keep your calories under 500.

Also, this form is very similar to the well-known "Eat-Stop-Eat" protocol, which is also discussed below.

Eat-Stop-Eat Protocol:

This particular form of Intermittent Fasting will ask you to fast for about 24 hours twice or once a week and it is strictly prohibited for you to eat anything during that particular period. And do the opposite during the other days.

To make things clearer, you can have your first meal at 7 AM on one day, then eat nothing until 7 AM of the coming day.

This particular program has been made famous by fitness Brad Pilon.

The 5/2 Diet:

This particular program asks you to eat healthy food for 5 days a week while making sure that you keep your calorie intake under 500-600 calories per day.

As for the fasting part, you are to simply fast for the next 2 days.

This particular form of fasting is extremely popular in America.

And just in case you are still not clear about the protocol, what you essentially have to do is eat on all days except for Tuesday and Thursday. On the alternate days, what you must to do is simply eat normally, making sure that you keep your calorie under a limit of 500 and break up those calories into small-sized meals.

The 16/8 Method:

The 16/8 method is the core method that I will be explaining throughout since this is often believed to be the most accessible and effective one.

This protocol is very simple as it will just require you to have a fasting window of 14-16 hours daily and have a feeding window of 8-10 hours.

It makes things easier for you, you can start off your day by having a meal at 8 AM in the morning, after which you may count 10 hours and keep feeding appropriately. Once you are done with that you will be too fast for the next 16 hours.

This cycle will keep on going. And just for the record, during your fasting window, you are allowed to drink "Zero Calorie" beverages like coffee or water.

Chapter 2 –Theory of Intermittent Fasting 16/8 and How It Works on Metabolism

Our diets in the modern world, beginning from about the nineteen fifties onwards, are packed with processed foods that turn healthy ingredients in our foods into unhealthy ingredients. That's right—the food packaging industry actually takes healthy ingredients and makes them unhealthy, without most of us ignoring why or how.

When it comes to fats, oils, and grains, the food industry encountered a crisis at the end of the twentieth century. Natural foods like dairy products and grains were going bad too quickly on grocery store shelves, and when food already has to travel long distances—this costs a lot of money.

So companies came up with two processes to chemically alter the ingredients in our freshest foods to make them last longer. Farming companies and packaging plants began running dairy products and oils through something called "hydrogenation." This process essentially warms the ingredients up to a hotter temperature to solidify the fat and oil molecules inside.

Grains undergo a process called "refining," where they're removed of things like a wheat germ that is good for our bodies but create shorter shelf lives. The result is hydrogenated oils, saturated and trans fats, and refined grains. These ingredients probably sound familiar because we're used to hearing about them often. Saturated fats are very unhealthy, as are refined grains and processed oilsbecause they raise our levels of bad cholesterol.

Cholesterol isn't just one number, which most of us think of because of the way cholesterol is taught to us. In reality, cholesterol is a fat-like steroid molecule that helps our bodies with plenty of tasks, but comes in both good and bad iterations. Processed ingredients like these three increase your levels of bad cholesterol by introducing low-density lipoprotein cholesterol into your bloodstream. Low-density lipoprotein cholesterol raises your levels of bad cholesterol, obviously, but it also actively works to lower your body's levels of helpful high-density lipoprotein cholesterol.

When we eat processed foods, the damage to our arteries is two-fold: your bad cholesterol rises, your good cholesterol lowers, and the result is a nasty build-up of plaque in the arteries around your heart. Remember that your heart is essentially a muscle. When plaque builds up in your arteries, your heart muscle has to pump that much harder to make sure the same amount of your blood gets pushed through a smaller opening. This causes your heart muscle to swell from over-work, and you can develop atherosclerosis—the pre-cursor to a heart attack.

There are two major explanations for intermittent fasting success.

They are periods of short fasting followed by periods of normal calorie intake.

1. This fasting method is that extremely low or no-calorie consumption is only done for short periods of time. A continued fast without returning to normal calorie intake will slow down the body's metabolism. However, short periods of fasting, like the 5/2 or 16/8 method appear to maintain and possibly increase your body burning calories.

Then, continuous fluctuation of fasting and normal food consumption, keeps your body on its toes, rather than allowing the metabolism to slow down.

2. Do not compare normal calorie intake to binging or excessive eating. What normal intake means is taking in what the body's approximate calorie needs is by eating a variety of healthy foods. It doesn't mean eating or binging on favorite foods that are unhealthy and have empty calories.

You may, after completing a fasting day, determined to continue consuming very low calories. This concept is very simple.

To keep the metabolism stoked and continue burning fat, your body needs a day of consuming a normal number of calories.

If you continue to maintain extremely low-calorie intake day after day without a break, your metabolism will slow down because the body will eventually go into a starvation mode.

However, when done properly, intermittent fasting seems to be reasonably safe, and could possibly be a better and more effective manner to diet, as well as improving your health.

Fasting and the Brain

Creates more brain cells. Fasting increases the rates of neurogenesis, which is the growth and development of new brain cells and nerve tissues, in the brain. Brain performance, focus, mood, and memory is connected to higher rates of neurogenesis. (Salcido, Dr. Brady, 2017)

Increases BDNF in the Brain. Fasting not only increases your rate of neurogenesis, but it also increases the production of BDNF, an important protein that has played a role in neuroplasticity and allows the brain to continue to adapt and change. The brain is much stronger, adaptable to change, and more resilient to stress.

The BDNF gene gives instructions for making a protein produced inside nerve cells. It produces new brain cells that protect your brain cells and stimulates new synapses and connections while increasing memory, learning, and improves moods.

Reduces Inflammation (Salcido, Dr. Brady, 2017). Intermittent fasting reduces inflammation. There are a number of ways for intermittent fasting to reduce inflammation.

Insulin Sensitivity

Fasting shows that it helps solve insulin resistance. Insulin and glucose build up in the blood and create inflammation when the body becomes resistant to insulin. Intermittent fasting gives the body a break. With no food to digest and the sugar stores are used up by the body, insulin levels begin to drop and lets the body re-sensitize to insulin again.

Ketones

While fasting, all the sugar stores are used by the body and have to turn to the fat stores for fuel. Ketones are created when fat is broken down. The ketones that are responsible for regulating inflammatory diseases like arthritis and Alzheimer's are B-hydroxybutyrate that blocks part of the immune system.

Autophagystimulates autophagy—so the body cleanses itself and reduces inflammation.

Burns Fat for Fuel

Surprisingly, fat is a cleaner and effective source of fuel rather than carbohydrates. Fat not only produces more energy per gram than carbohydrates do, but it can produce less free radicals, the cause of inflammation. When fat (ketones) or carbohydrates are used by your mitochondria, your cell batteries to make energy, there is a waste that gets produced which are free radicals.

The body goes through oxidative stress caused by free radicals, and is thought to be the cause of chronic diseases, including neurodegenerative diseases.

Boosts Your Energy

Intermittent fasting has been linked with the increase of mitochondrial biogenesis, the creation of new mitochondria. As mentioned, mitochondria are the batteries for your cells. Mitochondria fill each cell and power the cells to do their job. The cells' job is to take the food you eat and change it into energy. The brain gains more brainpower when you have mitochondria in the brain.

Boosts HGH Levels

HGH levels are naturally increased to give health, anti-aging, repair, longevity, and neuroprotective benefits by intermittent fasting. HGH can give neuroprotection, improve cognition, and increase neurogenesis.

Muscle Mass and Intermittent Fasting

Fat mass and lean mass will be lost when there is a loss of weight, and no exercise is included in a diet program. This is true of weight loss caused by both conventional diets and intermittent fasting.

Gaining muscle during intermittent fasting is another story. Research is very limited to whether it is possible to do so or not. This is probably because weight loss is the topic in most studies about these diets.

A study was conducted where a group of men were on a conventional diet or time-restricted eating program and completed a weight training program over eight weeks. Prior to the study, the group had not previously performed any weight training on a regular basis. During the study, the group was expected to eat all their food in a four-hour time frame, four days a week.

At the end of the study, the men who were in the time-restricted eating group maintained lean body mass, and their strength increased. The other group who followed the conventional diet gained five pounds of lean mass and also increased their strength.

The study showed that intermittent fasting is not best for muscle gain. It is possible that the time-restricted eating group ate less protein than the conventional diet group.

Other scientifically-based reasons are why intermittent fasting may not be ideal for gaining muscle. You need to eat more calories than you burn to gain muscle, consume enough protein so that your body can build new muscle tissue, and have an adequate exercise inducement to cause growth.

Additionally, in order to get enough protein, you may have to make a greater effort when eating less often than with a conventional diet.

All the reasons given do not mean that gaining muscle is impossible when following intermittent fasting, but it may not be easy to gain muscle. It is highly recommended that exercise, such as weight training while intermittent fasting helps in maintaining muscle, even when you lose fat. Additionally, other forms of exercise such as elliptical or a stationary bike may benefit maintaining muscle.

Weight Loss Through Intermittent Fasting 16/8

Intermittent fasting is proving to be a simple, convenient, and effective way to slim down. When done properly, it can result in positive changes to your body composition through loss of fat and weight. In today's culture, many people eat more calories than they burn in a day, which will lead to weight gain over time. When you better control your caloric intake, the opposite may be true. Caloric restriction and weight loss have been tied to a variety of health benefits.

Sustainable weight loss is often the main reason why people start on an intermittent fasting diet plan. Although intermittent fasting seems to offer the greatest benefits to those who are quite overweight, even if you only have a bit of weight to lose, you can reap many advantages from this change to your lifestyle. Intermittent fasting is a great way to kick-start your metabolism. It helps reduce body weight without losing any lean muscle mass.

Weight loss from fasting generally happens due to a number of related factors. To begin with, when you follow a fasting plan correctly, you should end up taking in fewer calories than your body is used to. Fasting should lead you to eat fewer meals than you normally would throughout a typical week.

Second, there are many positive hormonal changes brought on during a fasted state, most of which have already been discussed. Intermittent fasting helps optimize the release of two key fat-burning hormones, insulin, and human growth hormone.

The third reason that intermittent fasting encourages weight loss has to do with the positive influence that it has on your metabolism. Metabolism refers to the way your body converts food and oxygen into energy. Fasting increases your metabolic rates, which in turn helps your body burn more calories. Fat loss occurs when you burn more energy, then you take in. In order to lose weight, you have to do this consistently over time. Intermittent fasting works for weight loss by helping you eat less overall, and at the same time, burn more energy.

Fasting can also encourage fluid loss. The stored energy in your body contains a great deal of water. When you use up this stored energy during a fast, you are releasing a lot of excess water from your body. A positive side effect of this often reduced bloating.

One word of caution when it comes to this lifestyle plan. It is important to note that you are not likely to lose weight if you consistently overeat during your non-fasting times!

Chapter 3 – Potential Health Benefits of Intermittent Fasting 16/8

Weight loss and fat burning are some of the most talked-about health benefits of 16/8 intermittent fasting routine. However, the health benefits are simply not limited to weight loss. Intermittent fasting is a way to bring holistic health benefits.

It is a way of life that helps in improving the overall health biomarkers. You not only start looking fit from outside, but get fit from inside. It is a way to improve on many physiological parameters. It will help you in managing your blood sugar levels. It will also help you in dealing with your high blood pressure. If you are suffering from chronic inflammations, you will see improvement in it. If you have been struggling with cholesterol issues, intermittent fasting can help even in that area too.

Given below are some of the most important health benefits that can bring a positive change in your life.

Better Blood Sugar Control

Blood sugar management is directly related to insulin sensitivity. Apart from the people who are suffering from type 1 diabetes, most people face blood sugar management issues because their cells stop responding properly to the insulin signals. As a result, the blood sugar levels remain unreasonably high for longer periods; leading to several health complications.

However, insulin resistance is always at the core of this problem. If you want to have better control over your blood sugar levels, there can be no better way than intermittent fasting. It is the most reliable way to improve insulin sensitivity in your body. Your body will be able to lower the blood sugar levels faster, hence, you will be able to prevent a debilitating problem like diabetes forever. Diabetes never comes alone. It brings with itself several other health complications too. It is always best to keep this disease at bay.

Unfortunately, if you are already suffering from the problem, you must consult your physician before beginning intermittent fasting. People already suffering from diabetes would need a frequent dose adjustment of their medication, and also close monitoring of their blood sugar levels. Fasting for long can cause blood sugar levels to fluctuate at times, hence, it wouldn't be advisable to follow intermittent fasting without discussing it with your doctor.

Improved Heart Health

Every year, more than 635,000 people die of heart-related disorders in the US only. It is the number one cause of preventable deaths here. We all know that heart problems are a leading cause of death. We also know that most of us are likely to develop issues causing heart problems. Yet, we remain blissfully ignorant. Poor lifestyle, unhealthy choice of food items, and bad eating habits along with excessive stress, are the main things that cause heart problems.

However, we don't really do anything at all about most of these things. We keep blaming high cholesterol in our food most of the time for all the heart problems. Food manufacturing companies also keep marketing cholesterol as the main problem and never really focus on the real reasons.

Dietary cholesterol doesn't even constitute 20% of the total cholesterol in our body. Most of the cholesterol in the body is produced inside it.

The cholesterol is a building block for some of the most important hormones and also the cell structures. Without cholesterol, your heart may bleed to death. It is the main component that repairs the damage caused to your heart vessels.

Cholesterol is not the chief cause of the problems. Diabetes or high blood sugar can be the main cause, as it thickens the arteries and increases stiffness. The arteries are not able to expand when required.

High blood pressure is also a big reason for more heart problems, as it causes a lot of ischemic heart injuries. Your heart is pumping gallons of blood every day. During the course of its functioning, it keeps facing injuries. Whenever there is an injury, the cholesterol rushes to that part to mend the area which gets damaged. This repair and patchwork cause the heart vessels to thicken. Sometimes, the patchwork ruptures and forms blood clots that also cause blockages in the heart. However, cholesterol was never the cause of the problem in the first place. High blood sugar, high blood pressure, chronic inflammations in the heart region, high oxidative stress, are among the reasons that lead to heart problems.

Improved Mental Acuity

The brain is one of the most important organs in the body. It is crucial for our survival. We are called an intelligent race because of our developed brain. However, in the past few decades, there has been a significant increase in the cases of neurodegenerative disorders like Alzheimer's and Parkinson's disease. More and more people are getting affected by these problems, and the age of onset of these problems has also decreased. Meaning, people are getting affected by these issues quite early in their lives.

It is a condition that affects more than 5 million people in the US. Studies show that the risk of death due to this condition has increased by 89%. Yet, very little is done to prevent it. As per the experts, it is estimated that around 16 million people will be facing this condition by 2050.

The main cause of most neurodegenerative disorders is lower production of new cells. Like all other cells in our body, the brain cells also multiply, get old, die, and then regenerate. This keeps our brain forever, young and active. With age, people get smarter, sharper, and wiser. The process of the birth of new brain cells or neurons is called neurogenesis. For carrying out neurogenesis, a special type of protein known as Brain-Derived Neurotrophic Factor (BDNF) is required. However, oxidative stress, the presence of free radicals, and lower levels of antioxidants can lead to a decrease in the production of BDNF. It would also impact the process of neurogenesis and neuroplasticity.

Reduction in the Risk of Chronic Inflammations

Free radicals and oxidative stress are some of the terms you may be hearing a lot these days. The free radicals are nothing more than uncharged particles that haven't been used yet. Our body keeps producing free radicals as byproducts of various simple functions like cellular reactions, food metabolism, breathing, and other vital functions. Level free radicals don't pose any threat, and can also be used for fighting pathogens in the body or providing immunity. The antioxidants in the body maintain a balance between the free radicals and also prevent free radical damage.

However, over time, free radical damage can increase and may lead to chronic inflammations. Free radical damage increases when your body gets too dependent on glucose fuel as it releases a lot of free radicals. The greater the free radicals in your body, the higher will be the oxidative stress, and you would become prone to chronic inflammations.

Improved Satiety

One of the biggest problems faced by people suffering from weight issues is that they are never able to feel fully satiated from food. Although they may not feel significant hunger, they can't stop eating. Most of the time, this becomes a reason for social ridicule. However, it is not a thing to be laughed at. It is a physiological disorder caused by chronic inflammation in the fat cells, and it is known as "Leptin Resistance."

The hippocampus of the brain has the responsibility to receive signals from your body and transmit the message to you. For instance, when your fat stores get full, the hippocampus sends you a signal that you need to stop eating. You start feeling full all of a sudden. The gut sends the hippocampus ghrelin signals, and you start feeling hungry.

The fat cells release a hormone called leptin that sends the signal of satiety whenever you are full. When you are hungry, the leptin levels are the lowest in your blood, as they start rising as you start eating. The leptin levels would be the highest after 10-20 minutes of your full meal. It takes a while for your brain to receive the signal that your stomach is completely full.

However, you soon start to realize that the stomach is getting full, and your eating intensity and taste starts reducing. Sadly, that stops happening when a person is suffering from leptin resistance.

This problem is caused by inflammation in the fat cells. The fat cells start releasing leptin hormones at a steady rate. This means that in place of releasing the leptin hormone only when the stomach is full, the fat cells keep releasing it at a steady rate even when you have an empty stomach. This causes overexposure of the hippocampus to the hormone signal, and it stops registering the signal and reacting to it.

This means that you will never feel fully satisfied with food ever. Even when you have eaten more than required, you may not mind eating a bit more. This problem is more problematic for obese people, as they are never able to have any calorie restriction.

Intermittent fasting can help in resolving this problem slowly. When you fast for longer periods, the intake of food is stopped for long. The fat cells still keep releasing the leptin hormone, but the intensity never increases as the provocation of food is not there. This lowers the release of the leptin hormone. Slowly and gradually, the brain again develops sensitivity to the leptin signals, and things improve.

Who Should Avoid the Intermittent Fasting 16/8?

Intermittent fasting is a fascinating concept with great health benefits and the lowest risk factors. But it still poses a risk for some individuals. People with high energy needs, eating disorders, and diabetes shouldn't practice intermittent fasting.

People Falling in These Groups Shouldn't Practice Intermittent Fasting

Pregnant Women

Some experts say that pregnant mothers can practice intermittent fasting till the first trimester or can tweak the process a bit to practice it. However, pregnant women should not practice intermittent fasting at all in any form until they have given birth to the child and stopped feeding the child with breast milk. A pregnant woman has very high energy needs. She has to eat for two lives and even store continuously. Restricting diet at such a stage, or remaining hungry for long can have serious repercussions on the mental and physical health of the mother and the child.

Breastfeeding Mothers

If you are breastfeeding your child, then you should wait a little longer before you can begin intermittent fasting. It can cause severe energy crunch, as your body needs a lot of calories. You would need to eat at frequent intervals at this stage, and hence, intermittent fasting can be a very bad idea for you.

People With History of Eating Disorders

For obvious reasons, if you have ever had eating disorders, you shouldn't follow intermittent fasting, as that can trigger the same problems once again if they have subsided. Intermittent fasting can cause a severe nutrient deficiency in such people.

People With Type 1 Diabetes

People with type 1 diabetes should never practice intermittent fasting or fasting of any type for that matter. You would need to eat at regular intervals to maintain a healthy blood sugar level, and hence, you should completely avoid intermittent fasting.

Chronically Stressed People

Chronic stress can be a problem for a person trying to practice intermittent fasting. Food is deeply connected to our emotions and our sense of security. Prolonged deprivation of food may lead to mood swings and other similar problems. People with such a condition should avoid intermittent fasting.

People with Sleep Disorders

The toughest phase of intermittent fasting passes away while you are sleeping. If you have any kind of sleep disorder, then the chances are that it may get intensified due to the extra load of hunger pangs and food cravings. It may also affect your satisfaction levels. People facing such disorders should avoid fasting.

Chapter 4 –Longevity Enhancement

Researchers uncovered long ago that fasting is a way to promote durability in lifespan. A large section of information sustains the concept that limiting food intake reduces the danger of illness, usually in old age, as well as lengthens the period of life when invested healthily. Yet in the last few years, scientists have focused on this method of recurring fasting as an encouraging option to fasting. This means you do not require starving yourself to live longer always. The initial cross research between calorie limitation and periodic fasting was done way back in 1945 when it was found that recurring fasting extends the life expectancy of mice. Besides, there is research asserting that recurring fasting likewise decreases the danger of cancer, while at the same time enhances our cognitive feature. The theory behind this is that recurring fasting acts partially as a kind of mild tension that constantly revs up mobile defenses against molecular damage.

Prolonged Life Expectancy

Research studies recommend that periodic fasting might help animals live longer. As an example, one study located that short-term repeated fasting raised the life-span of female mice. The National Institute on Aging mentions that, even after decades of research study, scientists still cannot discuss why fasting may extend the life span. Therefore, they cannot confirm the long-term safety of this method. Human studies in the area are restricted, as well as the prospective advantages of periodic fasting for human longevity is not yet understood. The length of time prior to you seeing benefits of recurring fasting.

When it pertains to becoming healthier and toning up your body, one of the most preferred of the numerous choices out there right now is periodic fasting. Intermittent fasting includes numerous varietiesand approaches to select. Still, most involve eating for a short period of time during the day and restricting the number of calories you take in. The results appear to those who've tried the approach; however, according to the experts, you need a minimum of 10 weeks of complying with a few basic policies to see any modifications.

Illness Prevention

Advocates of intermittent fasting recommend that it can stop some problems and also diseases, including:

- Type 2 diabetes mellitus
- Heart conditions
- Some cancers
- Neurodegenerative conditions

Nevertheless, the research in this area remains minimal.

A 2014 testimonial reports that intermittent fasting reveals guarantee as an alternative to conventional calorie limitation for type 2 diabetic issues, aids fat burning in individuals that have overweight or weight problems. The researchers warn, nonetheless, that even more research study is necessary before they can get to reputable verdicts. A research study indicates that along with fat burning, an 8-hour eating window may help reduce blood pressure in grownups with weight problems.

Various other research studies report that intermittent fasting reduces glucose by 3 to 6% in those with pre-diabetes, although it has no effect on healthy and balanced individuals. It may additionally lower fasting insulin by 11-57% after 3 to 24 weeks of recurring fasting. Time-restricted fasting, such as the 16/8 techniques, might also aid grasping things and memory and decrease conditions that affect the brain. An annual evaluation notes that animal research has actually indicated that this kind of fasting reduces the danger of non-alcoholic fatty liver disease as well as cancer.

It Makes Your Day Simpler

In my individual experience, this is the component I enjoy the most (because I haven't lived enough time to experience what it suggests to live longer). It makes your day easier. I'm a huge fan of minimalism and also simplicity, and I choose to place my focus on many essential things in life. I delight in eating and don't mind not cooking; however, at the same time, I prefer to read, compose, make coffee, plan for my service, spend time with family, and also take some vacations. Obviously, I'm not the one who prepares seven meals a day for seven days a week, and I simply don't have time for that.

All that being claimed, the benefits of intermittent fasting go past simply weight loss. It additionally has many advantages for metabolic health and wellness, and may also help prevent chronic disease as well as expand life expectancy. Although calorie checking is generally not called for when doing recurring fasting, the weight reduction is primarily moderated by an overall decrease in calorie intake.

Studies comparing periodic fasting and constant calorie constraint show no difference in fat burning if calories are matched between teams. Intermittent Fast might help you hold on to muscle when weight loss sets in. One of the awful side effects of diet programs is that the body, tends to shrink muscle along with fat. Surprisingly, some researches are revealing that recurring fasting might be beneficial for holding on to muscle while shedding body fat. In one testimonial study, periodic calorie restriction triggered a comparable quantity of weight loss as continuous calorie limitation, but with a much smaller sized decrease in muscle mass. In the calorie restriction research studies, 25% of the weight shed was muscle mass, contrasted to only 10% in the periodic calorie restriction researches. Scientists have been researching periodic fasting for years. Research searching for is often inconsistent and inconclusive. However, the study on periodic fasting, consisting of 16/8 fasting, indicates that it might offer the following benefits:

Weight Loss

Eating throughout a set period can aid individuals to reduce the number of calories that they take. It may additionally assist in boosting metabolism. A 2017 research study suggests that periodic fasting brings about more effective weight management and weight loss in men with excessive weight than routine calorie restriction.

Chapter 5 –Troubleshooting During Intermittent Fasting 16/8

Now that you know all the ins and outs of intermittent fasting with the 16/8 method, everything will go perfectly. Well, in an ideal world, everything would be perfect. But as we know, nothing is so easy. Just like with any goal, especially for improving health, there is a high likelihood that you're going to run into problems. Once you hit a snag, it's easy to want to throw in the towel and just give up. But please don't. When it comes to following a specific eating schedule, it can be difficult, but the rewards are well worth it. So even if you're struggling, try to keep it up.

The Struggle

If you find that you're struggling with maintaining the fast, then there might be several issues happening. You might not be following a schedule that is good for you, or you might have jumped in too fast without giving your body time to adjust. Both things can make it difficult for you to excel at fasting. To help solve this problem, go back to your journal and see what you've done so far. Then change some things up. You could take a break from fasting and restart it, entering the fast slowly. You could also try shifting your eating and fasting windows. You could even reduce how much time you're fasting and just stay at 12 hours of fasting and 12 hours of eating for a couple of months. You could increase to 14 hours of fasting and 10 hours of eating once you are feeling more comfortable. Try different things to see what works best for you. Don't give up until you've tried a couple of different aspects.

Weight Gain

It's one thing to be working so hard on fasting, only to stay at the same weight. To gain weight while fasting can be really disheartening. However, don't take it as a sign that you should just stop fasting. You just need to tweak some aspects of your fast. There are many reasons why you might be gaining weight. Perhaps you may be eating too much, eating too little, or eating with poor nutrition.

Gaining weight from eating too much is self-explanatory. If you're consuming far more calories than you're using, then you're going to gain weight. When you're fasting, you may be eating more than you need for several reasons. Maybe you're subconsciously worried about going hungry, so to mitigate this problem, you eat a lot more for each of your meals. It's easy to see how this concern might lead to overeating. Instead of eating everything in sight, start paying attention to what you are eating and in what quantities. Keep a food journal or add a food journal to your fasting journal. Record everything you are putting in your body. When keeping a food journal, it can be surprising to see just what we are eating. We might think that all we had was a banana, but after reviewing the journal, we may see that we ate way more than just a banana. If you're someone who is an unconscious eater, someone who eats when stressed or bored, then you'll want to take a more mindful look at how you're eating.

After reviewing your food journal, look for areas you can improve. If you find that you're just eating massive meals, then find ways to cut down on what you're eating. You could replace half of your dish with a salad instead of more pasta, for example. This will help you feel full without ingesting as many calories as you would with a full plate of pasta. If you're worried about going hungry, how about trying to eat reduced portions first, then analyzing how you feel after. Do you feel hungry, or do you feel okay? If you are feeling hungry, then increase the protein and fiber in your meals. This can help calm your hunger hormone and make you feel fuller longer.

Another reason why you might be gaining weight is that you are eating too little. This sounds counterintuitive, but it makes a lot of sense when you understand the human body. When our body feels like we're not getting enough nutrition, it automatically decides that we must be facing famine. This is an evolutionary state where our body takes this environmental information and does everything it can to save us, even when we're not actually facing a famine. In order to save itself, our body starts hoarding everything that we eat and drastically reduces our metabolic rate, and if it's still not enough, it will start cannibalizing our muscles. In a situation like this, you would only lose weight once your body starts focusing on our slightly fewer necessary organs. In that case, you'll have a lot more to worry about than weight gain.

Keeping a Journal of Progress

Hopefully, by this point, you have a journal you're using to track your fast. The journal is awesome for keeping your fasting goals, having a record of your schedule, and tracking the success of your goals and diet. However, it can also be a record of your triggers and lapses.

Triggers are things that made you stop fasting or following your diet. People have different triggers, so it's hard to know for sure what will trigger someone to stop eating right or to stop fasting. Some examples might be a death in the family that causes you to lapse, or it could be a mental health difficulty that reoccurs and causes you to eat more than you should. If you're keeping a journal carefully, then you'll note times when you do not fast or times when you eat too much. When you see this pattern, try to understand what caused it. Was it something that happened that day that changed your mood, or was it something in your life that just made fasting too difficult at that time? Knowing what triggers your decision to stop fasting can help you either avoid it in the future or prepare a plan for when you'll be triggered again.

Lapses are very similar to triggers in that you choose not to follow the fast and stop eating healthily. However, these don't have to have a life event reason.

It can just be that you decided to stop. Maybe you were bored, or you wanted to stop fasting over the course of a vacation. You actively choose to stop, so this is a lapse. How you deal with the lapse can help you figure out how to avoid them in the future or how to shift your fast to better fit your plans.

Mindfulness

Often when we've gotten into the pattern of fasting or even just regular eating, we do so without thought. This often leads to overeating. It's been mentioned repeatedly that you should eat healthy meals in the right portions. The right portions are those that make you feel full without overeating or undereating. But what does that mean and what does that look like? We often don't recognize our own feeling of satiation until long past our overeating point. We also often miss our hunger cues or misinterpret psychological cues as hunger instead of listening to our body's hunger cues. This can cause us to struggle with our eating habits. To help us overcome this, we need to learn to be mindful of our eating habits and our relationship with food.

Mindfulness is the state of being aware of the present moment. It's about paying close attention to what is happening right now at this moment and allowing wandering thoughts to come and go without passing judgment. When it comes to eating, mindfulness is being aware of what is on the plate in front of us and being aware of our body's response to putting food in our mouths. It might involve paying attention to our five senses as we eat and taking the time to categorize what we're feeling. We might take a moment to understand where we are and what is happening around us. But then we always bring our awareness back to the food we are eating and our body's response.

The goal of mindfulness while eating is all about body awareness and food awareness. As someone who is already fasting, these are things you're already concerned about. Mindfulness goes into more detail about them. With mindfulness, you're learning to pay attention to your body. How does it feel as you are eating a certain item? What does the item look, taste, smell, feel, or even sound like? How does your body feel as the food goes down? And when you're digesting, what are you noticing? Has your energy level spiked or dropped? Is your heart racing or steady? Things like these are a part of mindfulness. These clues can help you know whether what you're eating is helping or harming your state of being.

With mindfulness, you're also learning to recognize when you are physically hungry, not just psychologically hungry. We can all look at the clock and say, "Man, I haven't eaten for hours! I'm hungry." But are we hungry, or is that just our psychological trigger telling us that we should be hungry? Learning to recognize our true physical hunger signs can help make the fasting process easier. It makes it simpler to know when it's time to eat during the eating window and when it's okay to continue fasting. Mindfulness can also help you know when it's time to stop eating. As we continue practicing mindfulness, you'll start to notice when your body becomes full and you are satiated. When you eat mindfully and slowly, this feeling will come earlier than you expect. This is because we often are too busy with our thoughts and activities while we eat that we miss the signal all too often. So mindful eating can change the way we approach food and change the way we choose to eat. It's a perfect solution to some of the difficulties with fasting.

Support Systems

The help that a support system can provide really can't be underestimated. When you're struggling with your fast, reach out to your friends, family, and loved ones. It's important to talk to people who will support you, not the people who will dramatically gasp, clutch their pearls, and scream that you're starving yourself. Talk to people who can help give you the motivation to continue fasting. You can even have friends who can help keep you accountable for following your eating schedule and eating healthy meals. If your friends want to join you while you fast, this is a bonus.

Some of us don't really have friends who can support us. In these cases, turn to social media. There are so many groups on Instagram, Facebook, or Twitter that are all about intermittent fasting. A personal favorite is the intermittent fasting group on Reddit.

Chapter 6 –Keep Track of Your Progress

If you are starting intermittent fasting not only to improve your health, but also to lose weight it is very important to take your initial weight, take measurements, and take pictures before you begin.

Scale Weigh-Ins

On the morning of day 1, it is important to get on the scale either nude or in very little clothes. It is important to weigh yourself before eating or drinking anything. Choose a time and weigh yourself, this will be known as your starting weight. It is important that you not only weigh yourself but also to write this number down and/or enter it into your phone or an app that you are using to keep track of your progress. I think it's better for you to write it down in a journal along the way so you can see your progress in real-time side by side.

It may also be a good idea to calculate your Body Mass Index (BMI) and your Body Fat Percentage, there are apps to calculate both, or a simple google search can result in free calculators to get this information. To prevent my scale victories from being non-victories, I choose the same day and time to weigh myself, once a week, only once a week. While intermittent fasting, you will lose inches faster than you will lose pounds from the scale, it is very important that you understand that, so that you don't get discouraged and quit. Therefore, I recommend not only to weigh yourself but also to take measurements and pictures to always see what progress you have made.

Measurement Tracking

On the morning of day 1, it is important to take your measurements. You will need to buy a measuring tape to have on hand. I purchased one in my favorite color to make me feel better about myself while taking the measurements. It is important to measure yourself before eating or drinking anything. Choose a time and measure yourself, this will be known as your starting measurements. It is important that you not only measure yourself, but also to write these numbers down and/or enter it into your phone or an app that you are using to keep track of your progress. I think it's better for you to write it down in a journal along the way so you can see your progress in real-time side by side.

I usually take the following measurements: neck circumference, waist, hips, arms, thigh, bust, belly pouch, and calf. You can measure more or less. I take 3 separate measurements from my waist and stomach area, because feel like its 3 separate body parts. I take measurements at the same time each day and week that I weigh myself.

Before & After

On the morning of day 1, it is important to take before pictures, so you have proof of how you looked on day 1. It is important to take your pictures before eating or drinking anything. Choose a time and get used to taking these pictures yourself, as someone may not always be around to help you with this (the same thing for your measurements, do this yourself), this will be known as your before picture.

I usually take pictures from all angles: front, back, both sides, one with a flexed muscle, etc., whichever pictures you decide to take do those same pictures each time you take pictures. This, along with how my clothes fit is all the evidence of what is really progressing and what is not or still needs work. Once, I have my pictures taken, I then use different apps to create collages to see the progress of the latest picture with the newest picture. I spend hours reviewing every inch of my body on these pictures to make sure I see all my victories. This is the best way to track your weight loss progress.

Main FAQ Intermittent Fasting

What's The Best Time for My Fasting Window?

Starting your fast as late at night as you can is the best way to maximize fat burn. Being active during the day while fasting will ensure you burn glycogen faster and move to fats earlier, so you have a longer fat-burning period. Starting your fast early on in the night will not help you as much as you are inactive and sleeping for most of the fast.

What Can I Do About Bloating?

Bloating can be a problem especially in the early days of intermittent fasting. Possible causes of bloating can be hormonal changes, increased water intake, and so many other reasons. Especially if your body is not used to drinking a lot of water, it will initially hold on to it since it knows it doesn't normally get enough. If this is the reason, then there is nothing to worry about as it will sort itself out as you go along. Another reason for bloating could be any food intolerances you might have such as dairy, gluten, etc. You can sort through this by a trial and error method by taking out one food at a time and seeing if it makes a difference.

Will Practicing Fasting Lead to Binge Eating?

Intermittent fasting need not necessarily lead to binge eating. But taking care to avoid a few common mistakes will help you overcome the urge to overeat. For example, break your fast with proper whole foods that keep you feeling fuller longer. Practice mindfulness to stay focused on your fast and keep motivated to stop yourself from breaking your fast or overeating. Start your intermittent fasting slowly and make it a point to eat well in your eating window.

Will Stevia Break My Fast?

Stevia is not true sugar, but it is processed and has calories and will break your fast. But it depends on how serious you are taking your fasting. If your intention in practicing intermittent fasting is healing and body cleansing, you will have to stay away from it. But, if you simply want to lose some weight and want a way to do that without the fuss of meal prepping, eating six times a day, while also being able to enjoy bigger meals, then stevia won't affect your fasts or stop you from achieving this.

Does Fasting Cause Muscle Loss?

No, intermittent fasting promotes lean muscle growth and only burns fats.

Do Calories Matter When Fasting?

There is enough research out there that supports both theories that total calories do matter even with fasting as well as the fact that weight loss is purely hormonal. It can be your own individual understanding. I believe in most cases calories do matter at least to some extent and if you eat more than you burn off you won't lose weight even if you fast.

Can I Apply Any Diet to Intermittent Fasting?

Yes, as discussed earlier, intermittent fasting is more a tool than an actual diet.

When is the best and worst time to train when following a 16/8 fasting schedule?

The worst time to exercise is the first few hours in the morning. Working out will cause hunger issues and since you have a few hours of fasting ahead of you it can make it more challenging. The best time to work out would be right before you are due to break your fast. And yet, if for some reason the only available time to you for workouts is early in the morning, then this is still better than not working out at all.

Who Should Not Do 16/8 Fasting?

Pregnant or breastfeeding women, women who are trying to get pregnant, people with type 1 diabetes, people with a history of eating disorders or are underweight, and individuals under 18 years of age.

People who are on prescribed medication, have gout or high uric acid, or people who have a history of or are currently suffering from liver, kidneys, or heart disease, are advised to stay away from fasting. If you have type 2 diabetes, you can probably fast but under a doctor's supervision.

What Side Effects Can Occur When Following a 16/8?

Common initial side effects include severe hunger, constipation, headaches, dizziness, heartburn, muscle cramps, tiredness, etc. Most side effects will disappear within a couple of weeks once your body adapts to fasting.

Can I Chew Gum While Fasting?

Yes, the effect is so small that it wouldn't affect your fast much. So, if you need to do that to get you through a fast, by all means, go for it.

Chapter 7 –Habits That May Increase the Efficacy of Intermittent Fasting 16/8

Intermittent fasting, even when using a mild program like the 16/8 plan, is a different way of living than most of us in the modern world are used to. That means there are going to be difficulties along the way and having a mindset for success is going to be necessary.

Food Is Not an Emotional Crutch

Many people use the consumption of food for emotional comfort. If that is something you're doing, consider leaving that behind. One of the benefits of intermittent fasting—provided you can follow it over a prolonged period—is that intermittent fasting resets your relationship with food. Some people aren't conscious of the central role that food plays in their lives. Of course, it's always going to play somewhat of a central role in your life, you have to eat to survive. But many people are actually obsessed with food, cooking, and eating. This can become unhealthy, even if you are not diagnosed with an official condition.

To Be Successful, Be a Member of a Team

It's hard to do anything completely alone in life. We all do better if we are sharing the experience with others and we are able to draw on the emotional support of others who are joining us on the same journey. This can be a problem for people with intermittent fasting, which the larger culture still looks at with a sideways glance. You might find that friends and family think you're becoming a little bit eccentric when they find out you're engaging in intermittent fasting. You might try explaining it to them and maybe even convince some friends and family members that it's completely normal and something that people should pursue.

Don't Let Setbacks Throw You off

Nobody is perfect and you can't expect yourself to stick to everything 100% all the time. Especially in the beginning, you are more likely to give into temptations that can cause you to fail when it comes to intermittent fasting. If that happens, it's completely natural. So, don't beat yourself up for eating outside of your feeding window or making other mistakes. A mistake is only a problem if you don't improve on the situation. Instead, you learn from it. Write down what you were feeling and what the circumstances were when you had your transgression. This will help you recognize when you are in a similar situation in the future, and then you'll be able to act with the conscious mind to prevent a second mishap.

Fasting Is Not a Quick Fix

Fasting is a lifestyle change that will lead to long term benefits. One mistake that people make is viewing fasting as another quick fix they can apply to their lives. It's understandable if you are impatient. Maybe you've been unable to lose weight for years and you're anxious to get started. The truth about intermittent fasting is that it's one of the most reliable methods if not the most reliable method for kick-starting weight loss and improving health. But that doesn't mean a magic genie is going to pop out of the bottle and give you instant weight loss. To be successful with intermittent fasting you should adopt a longer-term outlook.

Focus on Health First

Most people who are looking for intermittent fasting want to lose weight, and many want to lose weight to look better. Those are worthy goals; however, you will find you do better if you focus on health more so than anything else. The other benefits that come along will follow naturally if you are not so focused on your expectations of instant weight loss. Focus instead on improving your health, such as getting blood glucose and blood lipid numbers and reducing your risks of developing major diseases.

Recognize When a Fast Is Broken

If you are in the middle of a fasting period, and you have one bite of food, it's all over. That might sound harsh, but it's true. One bite is all it takes. Of course, we don't mean it's all over for eternity. What we mean is that your fast is over for that day. If you take a bite or taste of food and then "go back" to your intermittent fasting, the reality is you're not fasting. You can't consume any food whatsoever when you're in the middle of a fast.

You Don't Have to Tell Skeptics

You may have friends and family members who are skeptical about intermittent fasting. They may even think the idea is totally crazy. So why share it with them? If you are fasting, you don't need to tell anyone who isn't supportive about what you're doing. Remember, there are always online resources where there are people that can help. There is no reason to be talking to people that are going to be hostile toward your participation in this activity. In fact, if you are following 16/8 intermittent fasting, you don't need to tell a single person. It's an entirely flexible way to fast, and if you are meeting friends for dinner during your eight-hour window, they don't have to know a thing. You're the only one that needs to know about the eight-hour fasting window.

Set an Objective

One thing that is important for a success mindset is having a clear objective in mind. Before you adopt intermittent fasting, ask yourself what that objective is, and frame it in detail. If you belong to an online group, share it with them, and get them to hold you accountable if you aren't moving toward your objective.

Use Visualization and Meditation

Some people might think that visualization is fluff, but it can actually help keep you motivated. When you feel yourself feeling weak when it comes to meeting your health and weight loss goals, find a quiet space to meditate and visualize what the future will be like inside your mind, and picture yourself in a much healthier state due to the intermittent fasting lifestyle that you're using to reach your goals.

Don't Give in to Mental Fears

There is a lot of negative press surrounding ideas like intermittent fasting. But don't let those get to you. Intermittent fasting is perfectly safe and natural for most people. Don't let yourself internalize the fears and misgivings created in the larger society about intermittent fasting. The truth is people who are dead set against it probably don't understand it very well.

Use Affirmations

The mind has to be trained for success, and one of the most effective ways to ensure success is to train the subconscious mind. You can basically program your subconscious mind by telling it what to think. At first, this takes a large amount of conscious effort. But it comes down to a repetitive process. The more you repeat a thought or state of mind you want to have, the easier it's going to be to program the subconscious mind to adapt it. Develop a set of affirmations that you can say to yourself 2-3 times per day to get yourself committed to intermittent fasting. One important affirmation is going to be reminding yourself to not cheat when given the opportunity. Repeat this several times a day until you feel it flowing down into your subconscious.

Learn From Others

A decade ago, a person could be forgiven for going it alone with intermittent fasting. It was definitely fringe back then and it was hard to find information about it, much less talk to other people who had done it. Today, that isn't the case. Not only can you join message boards or Facebook groups to talk to others interested in the topic, but there are also plenty of blogs to read online and YouTube videos to watch. You can use these resources to learn from the experiences of others. This will help you see how others overcame obstacles, and you can learn what it feels like from others before experiencing it yourself.

Reward Yourself for Small Successes

To be successful, you don't have to reach your goals in one shot. When you are working toward your goal of incorporating intermittent fasting into your life, you may be at an intermediate stage and not quite there yet. Don't let that get you down and reward yourself for the progress you've made on your journey.

Get Plenty of Rest

Getting enough sleep is very important for overall health. Don't neglect this aspect of your health while you are engaging in intermittent fasting. This is very important when you are just starting out, and you might find that intermittent fasting leads to excessive fatigue, in the beginning stages. Getting proper bed rest will ensure your body is able to function at maximum capacity when you are adjusting to intermittent fasting.

Don't Give in to Fear

Fear should definitely not be an issue when using a mild approach like 16/8 intermittent fasting. But we are all human, and when you are in the midst of a fast you might find yourself questioning the process because of fears that rise up and grip you. If you experience this, consider reading to remind yourself of all the benefits of fasting. Keep articles and blogs that talk about the benefits of fasting bookmarked so that you can refer to them in your most difficult moments. Also, keep the reasons that you chose to follow intermittent fasting foremost in your mind, and remind yourself why you started fasting in the first place.

Focus on End Results

Think about how you managed to get through school or any other difficult task that you've done in life. If someone wants to get through medical school, one of the things they do to succeed and get through the hard times is they focus on the end goal. You should do this with fasting as well. If you are in the middle of a fast and the difficulties are starting to overwhelm you, focus on the end goal to help you strive to complete your fast.

With Intermittent Fasting, Realize Time Is Short

If you are doing an extended fast, it can be quite difficult to make it all the way. But the beauty of the 16/8 intermittent fasting method is that the amount of time spend fasting is actually pretty short, and you're going to be consuming food every day. You only have to get through a few hours, whether it's in the morning or at night before going to bed. Remind yourself of this when you begin losing motivation and you find yourself feeling that overwhelming desire to eat.

Don't Be Afraid To Get Help

As long as you're sticking to the fasting plans, you shouldn't run into any health problems. But if you do, don't be afraid to get help if you need it. Don't ever put your health at risk for the sake of avoiding embarrassment because you don't want those around you to know that you've been using intermittent fasting.

Chapter 8 –Planning Your Meals

Now we're at the part where we start to take action. I've told you about why intermittent fasting is a great option that you should consider, how this plan will help you, and how intermittent fasting should ideally be used in order to help you achieve successful weight loss results.

We are now moving on to the process of setting up a meal plan for the next two weeks. Even though we are only focusing on two weeks, this will give you a good taste of what intermittent fasting holds, how the program can benefit you, what you can do with such a program, and it will help you decide if this is an appropriate type of eating plan that you would want to follow.

Once you have completed the initial two-week period of intermittent fasting, you can decide if you want to go ahead and extend your program. At this time, you can continue with the plan that you have developed for yourself, or rather make some adjustments in order to better accompany your specific body and, of course, your goals.

Getting started is really the hardest part—and I believe that initial planning can really make things much easier. When you are organized and know what to eat and when to eat, you won't have to find yourself in chaos, unsure of what you will be preparing for dinner or any other meal. You will be able to have two stress-free weeks, knowing exactly how your day will go—at least in terms of food, that's it.

I am going to go through the process of setting up your intermittent fasting meal plan below. I will also provide you with some excellent recipes that you can follow. There are a lot of personal choices that will be implemented here, so the way you will be implementing an intermittent fasting program in your own life can likely defer from the next person's plans.

Understand Your Goals and Know What You Are Aiming For

We'll start off by taking a look at the goals that you are trying to achieve, what you are aiming for with the intermittent fasting diet that you are looking to start implementing in your life. Okay, I know—you picked this up because you saw that it is about using intermittent fasting for weight loss. You were not wrong, but the thing is, every person has different goals even when it comes to a specific topic like losing weight.

For example, a person who is obese will have to adopt a stricter diet and often include a larger caloric deficit, as well as understand that they will need to follow their diet plan for a more significant period of time, compared to someone who is only overweight and needs to lose just a few pounds.

Start by getting on the scale. Take down your current weight and consider your height—use a BMI calculator to help you determine if you are overweight, obese, or perhaps even morbidly obese.

Decide When to Eat and When to Fast

You now know your goals and have them written down, hopefully in the same file that you will be using to set up your intermittent fasting meal plan and track your progress. Before you continue with the process and start actually to set up a meal plan, we should first take one more step during the initial preparation phase—and this is to decide when you want to eat, as well as when you want to fast.

We are using the 16/8 intermittent fasting method. This means that for eight hours every day, you will eat. The rest of the time, which includes a 16-hour period, you will be fasting. Even though this sounds simple enough, simply stating that you are following a 16/8 intermittent fasting plan does not give you a view on when exactly each of these windows should be. At what hour should you start to eat and at what hour should your fast period start?

There are different ways to implement this program—but do not try to split the eight hours up. You cannot allow yourself four hours of eating in the morning, fast until four in the afternoon, and then have another four-hour eating phase. This will not work and is not how the program is supposed to be initiated. Your eight hours should be straight up—a single session of eating that expands over an eight-hour period in total for every 24 hours that pass by.

Calculate Your Ideal Daily Caloric Intake

Now we reach a very important part of your intermittent fasting program—calculating the most ideal number of calories that you should consume each day. In this step, it might also be a good idea to determine how many calories you'll have to burn. The data you calculate in this step will be crucial, as you'll have to fit in various meals into your daily plan assure that your intake of calories is not too high, but rather fits into your daily caloric intake goal.

This is also a step that can be difficult since there are a lot of mixed opinions on how many calories you should consume each day and how you need to calculate your ideal caloric intake for specific goals that you are striving toward.

In most cases, men are advised to consume a higher number of calories each day than women. These are the general recommendations for maintaining your weight (assuming you exercise enough to avoid a calorie surplus):

• Women: ~ 2,000 calories on a daily basis

• Men: ~ 2,500 calories on a daily basis

If 2,000 or 2,500 calories (depending on your gender, of course) is the recommended daily intake, then you would obviously have to lower this number in order to get to a daily caloric intake that will create a calorie deficit so that you can lose weight.

What to Eat and What to Avoid

Again, there are no rules on what you can eat and what you can't eat, it's a totally free choice when following the 16/8 diet. What you should bear in mind however is overall health and choices which are considered healthy, compared to unhealthy.

The idea is to create that calorie deficit during the full 24-hour span. You do this by ensuring that you fast and eat for the correct ratios of time, e.g. eight hours eating and 16 hours fasting, and that during your eating times you stick to healthy options as much as possible. You will feel infinitely better as a result.

If you want a few ideas on some of the healthiest foods you can incorporate into your day, check out the list below.

Eggs

Make sure you eat the yolk because this contains the vitamins and protein.

Leafy Greens

We're talking about things like spinach, collards, kale, and Swiss chard to name a few, and these are packed with fiber and are low in calories.

Oily and Fatty Fish, Such as Salmon

Salmon is a fish that will keep you feeling full, but it's also high in Omega-3 fatty acids, which are ideal for boosting brain health, reducing inflammation, and generally helping with weight loss too. If salmon isn't your bag, try mackerel, trout, herring, and sardines instead.

Cruciferous Vegetables

In this case, you need to look to Brussels sprouts, broccoli, cabbage, and cauliflower. Again, these types of vegetables contain a high fiber, which helps you feel fuller for longer, but also have cancer-fighting attributes.

Lean Meats

Stick to beef and chicken for the best options, but make sure that you go for the leanest cuts possible. You'll get a good protein boost here, but you can also make all manner of delicious dishes with both types of meat.

Boiled Potatoes

You might think that potatoes are bad for you and in most cases, they are, especially if you fry them, but boiled potatoes are actually a good choice, particularly if you're lacking in potassium. They are also very filling.

Tuna

This is a different type of fish to the oily fish we mentioned earlier and it's very low fat but high in protein. Go for tuna canned in water and not oil for the healthiest option. Pile it into a jacket potato for a delicious and healthy meal.

Beans and Other Types of Legumes

These are the staple of any healthy diet and are super filling too. We're talking about things like kidney beans, lentils, and black beans here, and they're high in fiber and protein.

Cottage Cheese

If you're a cheese fan, there's no reason to deny yourself, but most cheeses are quite high in fat. In that case, why not opt for cottage cheese instead? This is high in protein and quite filling, but low in calories.

Avocados

The fad food of the moment is actually very healthy and great for boosting your brainpower. Mash it up on some toast for a great breakfast packed with potassium and plenty of fiber.

Nuts

Instead of snacking on chocolate and chips, why not snack on nuts? You'll get great amounts of healthy fats, as well as fiber and protein, and they're filling too. But don't eat too much, as they can be high in calories if you overindulge.

Whole Grains

Everyone knows that whole grains are packed with fiber and therefore keep you fuller for longer, so this is the ideal choice for anyone who is trying intermittent fasting. Try quinoa, brown rice, and oats to get you started.

Fruits

Not all fruits are healthy, but they're certainly a better option than junk food. You'll also get a plethora of different vitamins and minerals, as well as a boost of antioxidants into your diet, ideal for your immune system.

Seeds

Again, just like nuts, seeds make a great snack, and they can be sprinkled on many foods, such as yogurt and porridge. Try chia seeds for a high fiber treat, while being low calorie at the same time.

Coconut Oil and Extra Virgin Olive Oil

You will no doubt have heard of the wonders of coconut oil, and this is a very healthy oil to try cooking with. Coconut oil is made up of something called medium-chain triglycerides, and while you might panic at the word triglycerides, these are actually the healthy kind. If you want to go for something totally low in calories, you can't beat extra virgin olive oil.

Yogurt

Perfect for a gut health boost, yogurt is your friend because it will keep you full and it also has probiotic content, provided you go for products which say "live and active cultures" on the label. Avoid both the sugary yogurt treats and anything that says "low fat." Normally, this isn't as positive as it sounds.

So, What Shouldn't You Eat?

There is nothing that is off-limits, but it's about how much of it you eat. If you want a slice of pizza, you can have a slice of pizza, but make sure you only have one and that you have a healthier diet for the rest of the day. Remember, one of the reasons why intermittent fasting is so popular is because it doesn't wag its finger at you when you grab a chocolate bar once in a while. You don't have to feel guilty because you gave in to a burger craving once a week, provided you know that moderation is the key.

Chapter 9 –Typical Eating Schedules for Intermittent Fasting 16/8

We've gone over the step-by-step process of transitioning into your fast. We've also looked a bit at making sure you have a clear record of the steps you are taking and how your body is adapting to the fast. Now let's look at some possible schedules for your fast. There is a schedule for your transition period and a schedule that examines what your daily eating times and windows will look like. Here are some additional things to keep in mind before looking at schedules:

Your Choice of Schedule Is Personal

Create one based on your work schedule or other circumstances in your life. If you want to have dinner with your family, then use that meal to close out your eating window. Count back eight hours to figure out when your first meal will be.

Your Fasting Schedule Doesn't Have to Be Set in Stone

Try out different times or change your fasting window for special occasions. You don't want to be limited by your schedule, especially when it comes to your social life.

A Great Option for Scheduling

To follow the times when you're naturally more awake and aware and end your fast before your natural slumps. Each person has a different internal clock, so determine your schedule based on that. Following your natural circadian rhythm is a good place to start; adapt from there.

Early Eating Schedule

This schedule is a great option because it takes advantage of your circadian rhythm. It also is the ideal time in general to eat because it avoids eating late at night. However, it means that you're going to eat an early dinner, which might not work for everyone. With this schedule, you'll start eating at 7:00 am and end at 3:00 pm.

Midday Eating Schedule

Some people have difficulty with eating first thing in the morning. In this case, you can start your fast later in the day. This fast is ideal for people who want to eat right in the middle of the day. It gives you time to wind down before bed and prepare your body for a time of rest without too much digestion happening while you sleep. It also gives you time to exercise in the morning before you break your fast if you want to.

Evening Eating Schedule

This schedule doesn't take advantage of your circadian rhythm, and it might not give you the most benefits in changing glucose and cortisol levels. However, this schedule can work for people who really appreciate social eating or people who work at unconventional hours. You can always eat a bit earlier to change this schedule.

These three different schedules give you some options for following your 16/8 fasting schedule. As mentioned before, adapt the programs to fit your daily rhythm and lifestyle better. It's ideal if your schedule is consistent, but it doesn't have to be set in stone. If you know you want to celebrate your best friend's promotion at the end of the week, then shift your fasting schedule to accommodate eating with your friends. Remember, fasting isn't a diet; it's just an eating schedule. It doesn't need to be permanent, and there shouldn't be any guilt about shifting your schedule.

Intermittent Fasting + Keto Diet: Should You Do Both?

Why is eating fat so good for losing weight? Fats, carbs, and proteins are known as the "macronutrients" and they affect our bodies in different ways. Fat by far is the most filling and calorie-rich food and helps us consume overall less daily by inhibiting the eating of other types of food. In fact, scientifically, one gram of protein or carbohydrates provides four calories, while one gram of fat provides nine calories.

A ketogenic diet is a high-fat, low-carb method of eating. (It is similar to the Atkins and low-carb diet, but critically different in this way.) Basically, by drastically reducing your body's intake of carbohydrates and replacing them with fat, you are putting your body in a state known as "ketosis." Although there are several variations of this diet, normally it consists of eating 75% fat, 20% protein, and only 5% carbohydrates. I will call these proportions the "standard" ketogenic diet.

There are three other types of well-known ketogenic diets:

1. The cyclical ketogenic diet involves having five ketogenic days followed by two high-carb days.

2. The targeted ketogenic diet (to be described here) is an adaptation that allows you to add carbs around your workouts.

3. Finally, the high-protein ketogenic diet is similar to the standard ketogenic diet, but includes a lot more protein. For this one, the proportions of the major components are 60% fat, 35% protein, and 5% carbs.

The ketogenic diet and the advent of intermittent fasting were first written about ancient Greek and Indian medical texts. Hippocrates' famous quote, "Let food be thy medicine, and medicine be thy food" was an early indication of the recognition and the importance of diet and nutrition on overallhuman health.The first study on ketogenic diets was done in France in 1911 on epileptics. At that time, epileptic patients were customarily given dangerous doses of potassium bromide, which resulted in major toxicity in the brain. They took 20 patients and gave them a low carbohydrate, vegan diet, and found that although only a few patients reduced their seizures, the majority of them had improved mental abilities. With the rise of allopathic medicine leading to the discovery of anticonvulsant drugs, these nutritional therapies were abandoned. But after seeing 20-30% of adult patients who were epileptic since childhood still with seizures in spite of the medication, the ketogenic diet was reintroduced, again with success. There is now no question the benefit of a ketogenic diet for childhood epileptic syndromes (such as West, Lennox-Gastaut, and Dravet) has been 30-40% effective based on current medical statistics.

Ketogenic diets have also been shown to help with Parkinson's disease, Alzheimer's disease, and dementia. Currently, researchers are looking at "ketone bodies" in the human blood and their health benefits. What they have found is beta-hydroxybutyrate (BHB), the most prominent ketone body, has the capacity to cross the blood-brain barrier and to be used for fuel for the brain similar to glucose or sugar. In fact, research has shown BHB to be more efficient (producing more energy per gram) than glucose. One medical doctor, Mary Newport, made the claim that she has reversed her husband's Alzheimer's disease using coconut oil. One of the main components of a ketogenic diet is consuming large amounts of fat, the most recommended fat being coconut oil. Large research studies are underway at major universities on the effects of coconut oil and mild chain triglycerides (a component of coconut oil) on cognitive function and impairment disorders. The results have been very promising.

What does this mean for intermittent fasting, ketogenic diets, weight loss, and performance? It means that if you follow these protocols, not only do you improve your physical health, but also your mental and emotional health. Hundreds and thousands of people have found relief and healing from many horrible illnesses and conditions by changing what, why, how, and at what frequency they eat.

In general, a ketogenic diet prescribes users to:

Avoid These Foods

Potatoes, rice, bread, pasta, cereals, grains, tortillas (flour or corn), fruit and fruit juices, soy products, fried foods, processed foods, refined sugars ("sodas"), chips and cookies, crackers and dips, alcohol, artificial ingredients, and artificial sweeteners. I know this sounds like a lot, but stay with me.

Stick to These Foods

Meats, fish, eggs, butter, nuts and seeds, coconut and avocados, cheese, heavy and sour cream, chicken and beef bone broths, low-carb veggies such as cauliflower, celery, onion, cabbage, bell peppers, squash, spinach, zucchini, and water, coffee or tea. Try to stick to organic, grass-fed, and cage-free products, if possible. It is best to stick to whole, single-ingredient foods for your meals. For instance, dark chocolate (~70% cacao) is a good treatment for people seeking to go into ketosis. Use these lists as a guide. There is "a ton" of information on ketogenic diets out there on the internet, including many excellent ketogenic recipes.

Similarly to intermittent fasting, a ketogenic diet has been shown to increase insulin sensitivity in the cells of the body, which lowers blood sugar. An advantage over traditional diets is its emphasis on the assimilation of fats of various types. Since intermittent fasting and the ketogenic diet have similar impacts on your body (getting it to use stored fat as energy instead of the food you just consumed) it only makes sense to try combining them.

If you are interested in trying intermittent fasting while using the ketogenic diet, keep the following things in mind:

Do Not Start Both of Them at the Same Time

Learn from the mistakes of others and from mine. Your body needs to get adapted to the ketogenic diet before it is required to go through long periods of time without eating. I recommend at first taking two weeks to get accustomed to the ketogenic diet without doing any purposeful fasting, and subsequently combine it with an intermittent fasting schedule best suited for you.

Start Out Slow and Go With What Feels Natural

You might automatically begin to detoxify or cleanse out in what is called a "Herxheimer reaction." Once your body adjusts to using up fat reserves and becomes "fat-adapted" you will start to feel less hungry. Try starting out by not snacking between meals before moving on to skipping a whole meal.

Keep Yourself Busy

Do not spend a lot of time hanging in and around your kitchen or supermarkets, and plan plenty of things to do to keep yourself busy. Do not surround yourself with temptation and get "out of the house" as often as you can.

Cook and Prepare Several of Your Meals in Advance

It's always easier to sit down and eat when you have prepared efficiently. Food preparation is much easier if you eat the same things three to four times a week. Getting a crock-pot was one of the best investments I ever made. Without much time involved, it helps me to cook lots of food, and I store it for later. One of my favorite cookware inventions of late is the Instapot.

Do Not Expect Your New Diet and Intermittent Fasting to Fix Everything You Might Be Ailing From

It definitely will help you lose weight and to be healthier. But, simultaneously, you should also be working on your stress levels and on getting enough sleep (you know when you need more sleep and it varies from person to person). And it's best if you can include purposeful exercise in your weekly schedule.

Chapter 10 –Breakfast Recipes

1. Choco Chip Whey Waffles

Preparation Time: 10 minutes

Cooking Time: 6 minutes

Servings: 2

Ingredients:

- 2 tablespoons organic coconut oil
- 2 tablespoons coconut sugar
- 4 tablespoons chocolate whey protein powder
- ⅓ cup almond flour
- A pinch of salt
- ½ teaspoon baking powder
- 2 eggs

Directions:

- Mix all the ingredients in the blender to obtain a homogenous paste.
- Preheat your waffle iron. Pour the waffle dough in the iron and cook each waffle for 3 minutes.

Nutrition: Calories: 423, Fat: 32.8 grams, Protein: 26.5 grams, Total Carbohydrates: 8.3 grams, Dietary Fiber: 2.9 grams

2. Coco Cinnamon-Packed Pancakes

Preparation Time: 30 minutes

Cooking Time: 5 minutes

Servings: 2

Ingredients:

- 2eggs
- 2½ tablespoons organic coconut flour
- ¼ cup milk substitute with hydrogenated vegetable oil (or almond milk)
- 1 tablespoon baking soda
- ½ tablespoon cinnamon
- ½ tablespoon baobab powder
- 2 tablespoons organic coconut flower syrup

Directions:

- In a salad bowl, mix the coconut flour, baobab powder, cinnamon, and baking soda.
- Add the beaten eggs, the almond milk, and the coconut syrup. Let the dough rest for 30 minutes.
- Cook the pancakes in a hot pan with coconut oil.
- Dress the pancakes with raspberries/blueberries or almonds.

Nutrition: Calories: 392, Fat: 32.5 grams, Protein: 20 grams, Total Carbohydrates: 11.3 grams, Dietary Fiber: 6.4 grams

3. Magdalena Muffins With Tart Tomatoes

Preparation Time: 10 minutes

Cooking Time: 20 minutes

Servings: 2

Ingredients:

- 2½ tablespoons whole-wheat flour
- 2½ tablespoons almond flour
- 1 tablespoon yeast or baking soda
- A dash of salt, pepper, and paprika
- 2 eggs
- 1 tablespoon organic cashew nuts
- 1 tablespoon hemp oil
- 2½ tablespoons soymilk
- ⅓cup feta cheese, diced
- 1⅓ cup dried tomatoes, without oil and sliced into small pieces

Directions:

- Mix the wheat flour, almond flour, yeast, and spices.
- Then add eggs, cashews, oil, and soymilk.
- Mix well to obtain a smooth paste. Add the feta and tomatoes.
- Mix well and pour the dough into muffin pans previously greased with coconut oil.

- Bake for 20 minutes at 350°F.

Nutrition: Calories: 405, Fat: 33.3 grams, Protein: 20.3 grams, Total Carbohydrates: 11 grams, Dietary Fiber: 4.9 grams

4. Spinach Shoots Mediterranean Medley

Preparation Time: 10 minutes

Cooking Time: 1 minute

Servings: 2

Ingredients:

- ½ cup spinach shoots
- 2 teaspoon quinoa
- ¼ cup avocado, sliced
- 1 teaspoon fresh goat cheese
- 1 teaspoon agave syrup, gluten-free
- ¼-cup dried blackberries
- 1 piece fig
- 1 teaspoon pumpkin seeds puree

Directions:

- Arrange the spinach shoots, cooked quinoa, and avocado on a large plate.
- Mix the goat cheese, agave syrup, and dried blackberries.
- Make 4 small cuts in the fig so that you can open it and insert the goat cheese mixture.
- Spread your fig on the spinach shoots. Sprinkle over with pumpkin seed puree.

Nutrition: Calories: 308, Fat: 26 grams, Protein: 15.4 grams, Total Carbohydrates: 9.7 grams, Dietary Fiber: 6.5 grams

5. Romantic Raspberry Power Pancake

Preparation Time: 5 minutes

Cooking Time: 10 minutes

Servings: 1

Ingredients:

- 2-tbsp raspberries, crushed
- 2-tsp almond flour
- 1-tbsp yeast or baking soda
- 1-tbsp vegan protein powder
- 2-tbsp soymilk
- 1-tbsp coconut oil

Directions:

- Mix the crushed raspberries and dry ingredients.
- Pour the milk and mix well to obtain a homogenous mixture.
- Cook the pancakes for 2 minutes on each side using a little coconut oil in a pan. Flip the pancake when small bubbles appear.
- Dress with almonds or nuts.

Nutrition: Calories: 323, Fat: 25.3 grams, Protein: 15.7 grams, Total Carbohydrates: 12 grams, Dietary Fiber: 3.8 grams

6. Chocolate, Chocolate Chip Muffins

Preparation Time: 10 minutes

Cooking Time: 11 minutes

Servings: 8

Ingredients:

- 1 cup almond butter, creamy
- 1/3 cup confectioner's erythritol (or preferred low carb sweetener)
- 2 tablespoons peanut butter powder
- 2 eggs, large
- 2 tablespoons cocoa powder, unsweetened
- 2 tablespoons filtered water
- 1 tablespoon salted butter, melted (or coconut oil)
- 1 tablespoon baking soda
- 1 ½ tablespoon vanilla extract
- ¼ cup dark chocolate chips for baking, sugar-free

Directions:

- Start by preheating your oven to 350 degrees F. set up a baking sheet with a mini muffin tin, silicone if you have it.
- Combine all the ingredients, except the chocolate chips, in a large mixing bowl, and mix together by hand or with an electric mixer. Make sure to blend all the ingredients thoroughly. The mix should be thick and doughy.

- Now add the chocolate chips and fold them into the muffin mix.
- Fill eighteen mini muffin or twelve regular-sized muffin slots about 2/3rd of the way full of the muffin mix.
- Set in the tray with the muffin pan on top of the oven and bakeat 350 degrees F for eleven min. When the timer goes off, take the baking sheet and muffins from the oven.
- To check if they are cooked through, use a thin knife or toothpick, and poke down into the center of a muffin. If the knife or toothpick comes out clean, then they are cooked!
- Allow your chocolate muffins to cool before enjoying them.

Nutrition: Calories: 100, Carbohydrates: 12 grams, Fat: 5 grams, Protein: 1 grams

7. Spinach and Mushroom Omelet With Goat Cheese

Preparation Time: 5 minutes

Cooking Time: 15 minutes

Servings: 1

Ingredients:

- 2 tablespoons olive oil
- 3 eggs
- 1 cup spinach
- 2 tablespoons goat cheese, crumbled
- 3 ounce preferred mushrooms, sliced
- ½ avocado, ripe and diced
- Black pepper and salt
- Fresh parsley, chopped

Directions:

- Heat olive oil in a medium-sized skillet on the stove over medium heat. Cook the mushrooms until they are tender and brown, this takes about five or six mins. Transfer the browned mushrooms from the stove to a bowl.
- Reheat the pan and coat with a little more olive oil. Whisk the eggs together and season with a bit of pepper and salt. Carefully pour the whisked eggs into the pan.

- Allow the eggs to cook until the edges start to set and the bottom browns. This will take approximately six to seven mins.
- Gently, using a rubber spatula, pull up the edges of the eggs to release them from the pan. Transfer them to a plate and lay flat.
- On half of the circular omelet set a layer of mushrooms, then spinach. Top with goat cheese and then the avocado slices. Fold the bare half of the omelet over the layered half and garnish with the fresh parsley. Enjoy warm!

Nutrition: Calories: 100, Carbohydrates: 12 grams, Fat: 5 grams, Protein: 1 grams

Chapter 11 –Snacks Recipe

8. Blackberry and Chia Seed Pudding

Preparation Time: 5 minutes

Cooking Time: 8 hours

Servings: 1

Ingredients:

- ¾ C almond milk, vanilla flavored, unsweetened
- 4 tablespoons chia seeds
- 3 tablespoons filtered honey
- 1 teaspoon vanilla extract
- 1 cup fresh blackberries

Directions:

- Mash up half a cup of the blackberries with a fork in a bowl. Combine all the ingredients together in a Mason jar, including the mashed berries, but excluding the remaining half cup of whole berries.
- Tighten the lid of the Mason jar and then shake the jar to get the ingredients well mixed and blended together.
- Let the Mason jar sit in the refrigerator with the pudding mix overnight.

- Scoop your pudding out of the jar and into a bowl to serve. Garnish with the whole blackberries that were set aside and drizzle with some extra honey or nuts as desired.
- Leftovers will keep when refrigerated for up to five days.

Nutrition: Calories: 323, Carbs: 6 grams, Fat: 31 grams, Protein: 5 grams

9. Carrot Sticks, Apple Slices, and Peanut Butter

Preparation Time: 10 minutes

Cooking Time: 0 minute

Servings: 4

Ingredients:

- 1 large apple
- 4 medium carrots
- Peanut Butter

Directions:

- Cut the apple in half and then slice each half into quarters, or sixths for thinner slices. Remove the seeds from the apple slices.
- Cut the carrots in half and then cut the halves into thirds or quarters, depending on the desired slice thickness.
- Dip the apple slices and carrot sticks into peanut butter liberally and enjoy it! A great snack for around the house or at work.

Nutrition: Calories: 130, Carbs: 25 grams, Fat: 4 grams, Protein: 2 grams

10.   Fruit and Cheese Plate

Preparation Time: 5 minutes

Cooking Time: 0 minute

Servings: 4

Ingredients:

- Red Grapes
- Green Grapes
- One Pear
- Cherries
- Cheddar Cheese
- Gouda Cheese
- Brie Cheese
- Quinoa Crackers

Directions:

- Cut the pear in half and then slice the halves into four to six thinner slices. Remove the seeds.
- Cut the cheddar, gouda, and brie cheese into square slices. Make them as thick or thin as you'd like.
- Arrange the fruits and cheeses on a plate with the quinoa crackers. Enjoy with family and friends. Or pack up in a travel container and bring to work as a snack between meals.

Nutrition: Calories: 240, Carbs: 15 grams, Fat: 2 grams, Protein: 8 grams, Fiber: 3 grams

11.   Trail Mix

Preparation Time: 2 minutes

Cooking Time: 0 minute

Servings: 1

Ingredients:

- 1 cup almonds, roasted
- ½ cup cashews
- ½ cup sunflower seeds
- ¼ cup coconut, shredded
- Handful dried cranberries

Directions:

- Combine all ingredients in a jar or container with a lid.
- Shake the container to mix the ingredients together.
- Store in an airtight, glass container.
- A single portion is about one handful of the mix.

Nutrition: Calories: 160, Carbs: 14 grams, Fat: 9 grams, Protein: 5 grams

12.   Cheese Mug

Preparation Time: 4 minutes

Cooking Time: 1 to 2 minutes

Servings: 1

Ingredients:

- 2 ounces roast beef slices
- 1 and ½ tablespoons green chilies, diced
- 1 and ½ ounces pepper jack cheese, shredded
- 1 tablespoon sour cream

Directions:

- Layer roast beef on the bottom of your mug, making sure to break it down into small pieces.
- Add half a tablespoon of sour cream, add half tablespoon green Chile and half an ounce of pepper jack cheese.
- Keep layering until all ingredients are used.
- Microwave for 2 minutes.
- Serve warm and enjoy!

Nutrition: Calories: 268, Fat: 16 grams, Carbohydrates: 4 grams, Protein: 22 grams

13.   Lemon Broccoli

Preparation Time: 10 minutes

Cooking Time: 15 minutes

Servings: 4

Ingredients:

- 2 heads broccoli, separated into florets
- 2 teaspoons extra virgin olive oil
- 1 teaspoon salt
- ½ teaspoon pepper
- 1 garlic clove, minced
- ½ teaspoon lemon juice

Directions:

- Preheat your oven to a temperature of 400 degrees F.
- Take a large-sized bowl and add the broccoli florets with some extra virgin olive oil, pepper, sea salt and garlic.
- Spread the broccoli out in a single evenly layer on a fine baking sheet.
- Bake in your pre-heated oven for about 15-20 minutes until the florets are soft enough so that they can be pierced with a fork.
- Squeeze lemon juice over them generously before serving.

Nutrition: Calories: 49, Fat: 2 grams, Carbohydrates: 4 grams, Protein: 3 grams

14.   Coconut Candy

Preparation Time 10 minutes

Cooking Time: 0 minutes

Servings: 1

Ingredients:

- 2-tbsp coconut butter (or notably known as Coconut Manna)

Directions:

- Melt the coconut butter at room temperature until it resembles a creamy butter consistency.
- Spoon out the melted butter into candy molds. Refrigerate for 10 minutes to harden before serving.

Nutrition: Calories: 204, Fat: 17.2 grams, Protein: 10.2 grams, Carbohydrates: 3 grams, Fiber: 0.8 grams

Chapter 12 –Main Meals

15.   Pizza Pie with Cheesy Cauliflower Crust

Preparation Time: 5 minutes

Cooking Time: 30 minutes

Servings: 2

Ingredients:

- ½ head cauliflower, rinsed, riced, cooked for 5 minutes in boiling water, and drained
- 2eggs, whisked
- ⅓Parmesan cheese
- ½ cup cherry tomatoes, washed and halved
- 2 tablespoon organic hempseed oil
- 1 teaspoon balsamic vinegar
- 1 mozzarella cheese ball, crumbled
- ¼ cup basil leaves

Directions:

- Spin the cooked cauliflower in a dishtowel to let out as much liquid as possible. (The goal is to obtain a floury texture.) Add the eggs and cheese. Mix well.

- Spread to a disk the cauliflower dough on a baking pan lined with parchment paper. Bake for 15 minutes at 400°F in your preheated oven.
- Meanwhile, mix the tomatoes with hempseed oil and balsamic vinegar. Season the mixture with salt and pepper.
- Remove the pizza dough from the oven. Add the tomato mixture and sprinkle over with mozzarella. Return the pan in the oven and bake further for 15 minutes.
- Serve hot and garnish with fresh basil leaves.

Nutrition: Calories: 384, Fat: 32 grams, Protein: 20 grams, Total Carbohydrates: 6 grams, Dietary Fiber: 2grams

16.   Roasted Rib-Eye Skillet Steak

Preparation Time: 5 minutes

Cooking Time: 15 minutes

Servings: 2

Ingredients:

- 1-16 ounce rib-eye steak (1 to 1¼-inch thick)
- 2 tablespoon duck fat or peanut oil (divided)
- A dash of salt and pepper
- 1 tablespoon butter
- ½ teaspoon thyme, chopped

Directions:

- Preheat your oven to 400°F. Place a cast-iron skillet inside.
- Season the rib-eye steak with oil, salt, and pepper.
- Take the preheated skillet out from the oven and place over the stove, set in medium heat. Pour oil, and add the steak. Sear for 2 minutes on both sides.
- Return the skillet with the steak in the oven. Roast for 6 minutes.
- Remove the skillet and place over the stove, set on low heat. Add the butter and thyme in the skillet. Baste the steak for about 4 minutes.

Nutrition: Calories: 722, Fat: 60 grams, Protein: 45 grams, Total Carbohydrates: 0 gram, Dietary Fiber: 0 gram

17.   Spaghetti With Asian Sauce

Preparation Time: 10 minutes

Cooking Time: 15 minutes

Servings: 2

Ingredients:

- For the Sauce:
- 2 teaspoons soy sauce, gluten-free
- 1 teaspoon of hemp oil
- 1 teaspoon of lemon juice
- 1 tablespoon peanut butter
- For the Spaghetti:
- ½-bulb onion, diced
- 1 teaspoon coconut oil
- 1 teaspoon red or green pepper, diced
- 1 piece carrot, thinly sliced lengthwise
- 1 egg, whisked
- 5-oz. low-carb spaghetti, rinsed and cooked for 2 minutes in boiling water
- Fresh coriander and peanuts for garnish

Directions:

- Combine all the sauce ingredients in a bowl. Set aside.
- Sauté the onion with oil, and add the peppers, carrots, egg, sauce, and spaghetti. Cook for 13 minutes, stirring frequently.

- To serve, garnish with fresh coriander and peanuts.

Nutrition: Calories: 412, Fat: 34.4 grams, Protein: 20.9 grams, Total Carbohydrates: 10.5 grams, Dietary Fiber: 5.7 grams

18. Shirataki & Soy Sprouts Pad Thai With Peanut Tidbits

Preparation time: 10 minutes

Cooking Time: 5 minutes

Servings: 1

Ingredients:

For the Sauce:

- 1 tablespoon peanut butter
- 2 tablespoons soy sauce, gluten-free
- ½ lime
- 2 tablespoon agave syrup, gluten-free
- ½ tablespoon organic turmeric

For the Noodles:

- 1 bag of konjac shirataki noodles, rinsed and cooked for 2 minutes in boiling water
- 1 piece carrot, thinly sliced
- 1-bulb onion, thinly sliced
- ½-cup soy sprouts
- ¼-cup unsalted peanuts
- Some sprigs of fresh coriander

Directions:

- Combine all the sauce ingredients in a bowl. Set aside.

- Heat the pasta with a little coconut oil in a frying pan. Pour the sauce and add the coriander. Mix well and cook for 5 minutes.
- To serve, place in a bowl and garnish with peanuts and coriander sprigs.

Nutrition: Calories: 423, Fat: 35.2 grams, Protein: 21 grams, Total Carbohydrates: 14.9 grams, Dietary Fiber: 9.6 grams

19. Charred Chicken with Squash Seed Sauce

Preparation Time: 15 minutes

Cooking Time: 20 minutes

Servings: 1

Ingredients:

For the Sauce:

- 2 tablespoons white almond puree
- 2-cloves of garlic, finely chopped (divided, for the sauce and chicken marinade)
- ½ tablespoon squash seeds
- 1 tablespoon barley
- 1 piece fresh basil

For the Marinade:

- 2 branches rosemary, finely chopped
- 1 piece red chili, finely chopped
- 1 piece lemon (keep the zest)
- Pinch of salt and ground black pepper
- 1 tablespoon olive oil
- 1 cup chicken breasts, cubed
- 5 bulbs small onions, sliced in quarters
- 5 pieces cherry tomatoes

Directions:

- Combine and mix all the sauce ingredients in a bowl. Set aside.
- Mix all the marinade ingredients and let stand for 10 minutes. Thread alternately the onions, meat, and tomatoes onto the skewers and grill over a coal fire for 10 minutes on each side. Serve the chicken kebabs with the squash seed sauce.

Nutrition: Calories: 428, Fat: 35.6 grams, Protein: 21 grams, Total Carbohydrates: 16.9 grams, Dietary Fiber: 11.6 grams

20.   Meatballs and Pasta with Sauce

Preparation Time: 20 minutes

Cooking Time: 15 minutes

Servings: 4

Ingredients:

For Meatballs:

- 1 pound beef, ground
- ½ cup mozzarella cheese, shredded
- ¼ cup parmesan cheese, grated
- 1 minced garlic clove
- 1 egg, large and beaten
- 2 tablespoons fresh parsley, chopped
- ½ teaspoon black pepper, freshly ground
- 1 teaspoon salt
- 2 tablespoons olive oil

For Sauce:

- 28 ounces tomatoes, canned and crushed
- 1 chopped onion
- 1 teaspoon oregano, dried
- 2 minced garlic gloves
- Salt and pepper
- For Spaghetti:
- 1 medium spaghetti squash
- Olive oil

- Salt and pepper

Directions:

- Preheat the oven to 350 degrees F. Cut the spaghetti squash in half and spoon out the seeds, leaving as much of the flesh intact as possible. Brush the halves with olive oil and season with salt and pepper. Set the squash halves to face down on a baking sheet.
- Bake the squash for thirty to forty minutes.
- While the squash is baking, assemble the meatballs. Combine together the beef, cheeses, egg, garlic, parsley, and the salt and pepper. Mix the ingredients together well and then form sixteen meatballs by hand.
- Set a burner to medium heat and place a skillet over the burner. Heat the olive oil and then put the meatballs into the skillet. Turn them occasionally until the meatballs have become golden on all sides. It should take about ten mins.
- Remove the meatballs from the heat when they are golden and set on a plate that is lined with a paper towel.
- Use the same skillet to make the sauce. Soften the onion for five mins. Add in the garlic and sauté until deliciously fragrant, about one min. Mix the tomatoes, salt, pepper, and oregano into the pot.

- Once stirred, throw the meatballs back in the skillet with the sauce. Cover the pot and let the sauce and meatballs simmer for fifteen mins for the sauce to thicken.
- When the spaghetti squash is done in the oven, poke it with a fork to make sure it is tender. Allow cooling until it can be handled. Then use a fork to scrape out the flesh of the squash, and it will shred into squash noodles.
- Divide the squash noodles onto plates and top with scoops of sauce and meatballs. Sprinkle with a little parmesan cheese and then serve!

Nutrition: Calories: 165, Carbohydrates: 7 grams, Fat: 0 gram, Protein: 1 grams

21.   Grilled Salmon, Veggies, and Rice

Preparation Time: 5 minutes

Cooking Time: 10 minutes

Servings: 4

Ingredients:

- Salmon
- 1 ½ pound salmon, sliced into 4 smaller fillets
- Olive oil
- ¼ cup of salt
- ¼ cup onion powder
- ¼ cup basil
- ¼ cup garlic powder
- ¼ cup dried parsley
- 2 zucchinis halved and then quartered the long way
- 2bell peppers, quartered
- 1 summer squash halved and then quartered the long way
- 1 ½ cup Jasmine Rice
- 3 cups of water

Directions:

- To make the seasoning, mix all the seasoning ingredients together and blend evenly. Store the seasoning in an airtight jar for as much as six months.

- Rub the olive oil into each salmon filet, on both sides. Sprinkle the fillets with some of the seasonings, depending on your own flavor pallet.
- Skewer the vegetable chunks onto wooden or metal kabob skewers.
- Heat the goals on your grill, or set a gas grill to medium heat. Set the salmon directly on the grill grate. Close the grill id and cook the fish for about five min. on each side. Turn the vegetable skewers every few minutes for even heating.
- When the salmon is flaky, it is ready to come off the grill. When the veggies are tender and are starting to get brown spots, they are ready to come off the grill.
- On the stove, heat the three cups of water in a medium saucepan until boiling. Add the jasmine rice, sprinkle in a little salt, and stir the rice.
- Lower the heat on the stove down to a low simmer and cover the rice. Allow the water to simmer off and the rice to cook about fifteen to twenty minutes.
- When the rice is finished, divide onto four plates. Top the rice with salmon and serve with grilled veggies on the side.

Nutrition: Calories: 420, Carbohydrates: 5 grams, Fat: 31 grams, Protein: 35 grams

Conclusion

Thank you for making it to the end. There are plenty of diets out there, all promising you the impossible. Incredible weight loss, with no mention of any side effects, you are probably fed up with the "lose x pounds in 30 days, guaranteed" approach. Many of these diets are not backed up by science, or in other words, there is not any scientific research to prove these diets actually deliver what they promise. They focus only on the weight loss process, suggesting meal plans that are extremely radical in some cases.

At the end of this book, the main benefits of intermittent fasting can be summarized in 8 points:

- Eliminates precancerous and cancerous cells
- Shifts easily into nutritional ketosis
- Reduces the fat tissue
- Enhances the gene expression for healthspan and longevity
- Induces autophagy and the apoptotic cellular repair or cleaning
- Improves your insulin sensitivity

- Reduces inflammation and oxidative stress

- Increases neuroprotection and cognitive effects

To expand on the benefits of this practice, intermittent fasting can have positive impacts over the fat loss process, disease prevention, anti-aging, therapeutic benefits (psychological, spiritual and physical), mental performance, physical fitness (improved metabolism, wind, and endurance, the great effect over bodybuilding).

As you restrain yourself from eating, the body will no longer have available glucose to use in order to produce energy. Therefore, it will use ketones to break the fat tissue open and release the energy stored in there. This is how the body will burn your existing fat in order to generate energy. When it comes to diets, they are not designed for the long run, and as soon as you break the diet, you will start gaining weight again. Intermittent fasting is something that you can try for a lifetime because it is easy to stick to it, and it doesn't involve any special meal plan. So, you can still eat your favorite foods, as long as you schedule your meals, allowing a smaller eating window and a longer fasting period. IF induces ketosis and eventually autophagy, which will definitely mean reducing the fat reserves.

Do you know that intermittent fasting is, in fact, a cure for several different diseases and medical conditions? You would definitely become more interested in this process. There are a few studies that show the beneficial effects IF has on your health. A study published in the World Journal of Diabetes has shown that patients with type 2 diabetes on short-term daily intermittent fasting experience a lower body weight, but also a better variability of post-meal glucose.

Other benefits this diet has:

- Enhances the markers of stress resistance
- Reduces the blood pressure and inflammation
- Better lipid levels and glucose circulation, which may lead to a lower risk of cardiovascular disease, neurological diseases like Parkinson's and Alzheimer's, and also cancer

Take note that the modern-day lifestyle includes too much stress and is too sedentary. Whether we like it or not, these factors have a great contribution to the aging process. You are probably wondering what intermittent fasting can do the slow down this process, as we all know that it can't be stopped. IF is not "the fountain of youth" and it will not grant you immortality, but it can still lower the blood pressure and reduce oxidative damage, enhance your insulin sensitivity and reduce your fat mass. Coincidence or not, all of these factors are known to improve your health and longevity. Intermittent fasting is one of the triggering factors of autophagy, a process known for destroying and replacing old cell parts with new ones, at any level within your body. Such a process can slow down the aging process.

I hope you learned something!

Did you enjoy this book?

If you enjoyed this book, it would be awesome if you could leave a quick review on Amazon. Your feedback is much appreciated and I would love to hear from you.

<u>Leave a Review on Amazon</u>

Thanks so much!!

More books by Geena Moore:

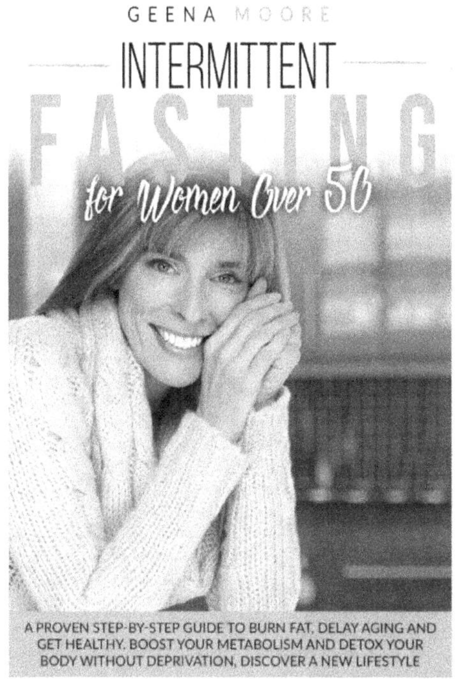

Intermittent Fasting for Women Over 50: A Proven Step-By-Step Guide to Burn Fat, Delay Aging and Get Healthy. Boost Your Metabolism and Detox Your Body without Deprivation, Discover a New Lifestyle. (Link)

More books by Geena Moore:

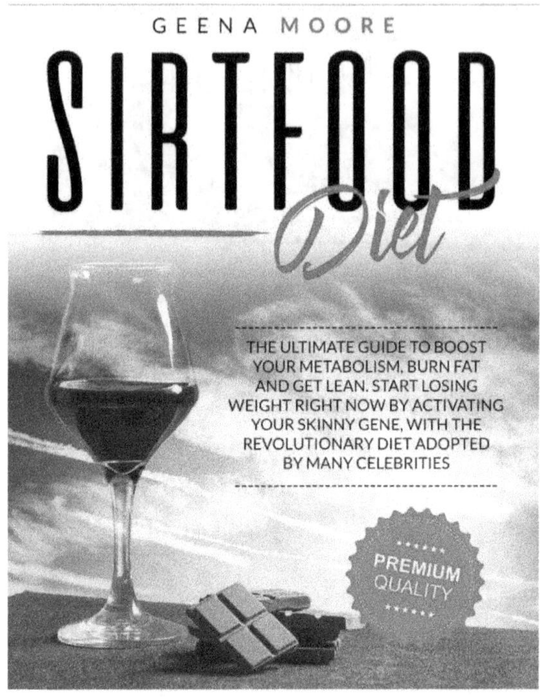

Sirtfood Diet: The Ultimate Guide to Boost YOUR Metabolism, Burn Fat and Get Lean. Start Losing Weight RIGHT NOW by Activating Your Skinny Gene with the Revolutionary Diet Adopted by Many Celebrities. (Link)

More books by Geena Moore:

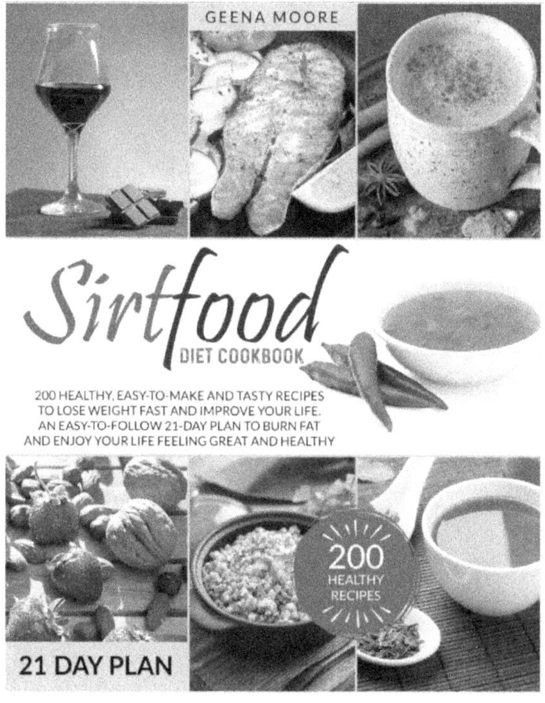

Sirtfood Diet Cookbook: 200 Healthy, Easy-To-Make and Tasty Recipes to Lose Weight Fast and Improve YOUR Life. An Easy-To-Follow 21-Day Plan to Burn Fat and Enjoy YOUR Life Feeling Great and Healthy. (Link)

9 798559 195070